# Facing Learning Disabilities in the Adult Years

# Facing Learning Disabilities in the Adult Years

JOAN SHAPIRO

REBECCA RICH

*New York  Oxford*
OXFORD UNIVERSITY PRESS
1999

Oxford University Press

Oxford    New York

Athens    Auckland    Bangkok    Bogotá    Bombay
Buenos Aires    Cape Town    Chennai    Dar es Salaam
Delhi    Florence    Hong Kong    Istanbul    Karachi
Kuala Lumpur    Madrid    Melbourne    Mexico City
Mumbai    Nairobi    Paris    São Paulo    Singapore
Taipei    Tokyo    Toronto    Warsaw

and associated companies in
Berlin    Ibadan

Published by Oxford University Press, Inc.
198 Madison Avenue, New York, New York 10016

Oxford is a registered trademark of Oxford University Press

Library of Congress Cataloging-in-Publication Data
Shapiro, Joan (Joan M.)
Facing learning disabilities in the adult years / Joan Shapiro, Rebecca Rich.
p.  cm.    Includes bibliographical references (p.  ) and index
ISBN 0-19-511335-7
1. Learning disabilities—United States.
I. Rich, Rebecca (Rebecca Z.)    II. Title.
LC4818.5.S53    1999    371.9'0475—dc21    99-29267

9 8 7 6 5 4 3 2 1

Printed in the United States of America
on acid-free paper

*This book is dedicated to our families,*
*who have always been a great source*
*of support and encouragement.*

❖   ❖   ❖

Our thanks to production editor Joellyn Ausanka and the editorial staff for all their help. Our special thanks to Joan Bossert, who encouraged our work from the outset. It was a pleasure to have the opportunity to work with her. Her guidance and support were invaluable, as was her judgment in steering us in the right direction.

We extend our appreciation to all the adults who were so willing to share their experiences and a special thanks to Michael Trotta for offering us his story and written material.

# Contents

# Facing Learning Disabilities
# in the Adult Years

# 1

## *Introduction*

At twenty-seven, Jennifer feels successful for the first time in her life. Ten years ago, she dropped out of high school: "I was competent socially. I was a cheerleader, had lots of friends, both male and female, and, overall, was very popular. But going to classes was a nightmare. So I avoided schoolwork and instead spent all my time socializing and getting into trouble. Finally, I couldn't take the failure and disapproval of my parents, my teachers, and even some of my classmates, and I left school. My parents were shocked, as everyone in my family had gone to college."

After working for several years at low-paying jobs, Jennifer earned a high school equivalency degree. She then enrolled in a college, but did poorly and was dismissed. Two years ago, Jennifer tried another college, this time one with a support program designed for students with learning disabilities. To her delight and surprise, she is maintaining a B average: "I am working hard, harder than I have ever worked in my life. But I see the results of my efforts. I feel so good. I wish I could go back and tell some of my former teachers and classmates, 'You were all wrong. I really am not stupid.'"

This book is about adults, like Jennifer, who have learning disabilities. As educators, we have been impressed by the increased numbers of adults with learning disabilities looking for answers and help. They range in age from twenty to sixty, but their questions are the same: What is a learning disability? Can I get help at my age? What type of help is available? Should I give up my goals? What is the next step? Most adults talk about their past and present struggles in school or on the job. They are eager to come to terms with the disability that, in many cases, has never been diagnosed, treated, or even explained to them.

Who are these adults? The single label, *learning disability*, belies the

[3]

fact that there is an enormous range of abilities, needs, and patterns of strengths and weaknesses unique to each individual. Some adults with learning disabilities adjust very well to the different stages and problems that are part of adult life. They acquire and maintain good jobs, get promoted, participate in community activities, and have satisfying personal relationships. Others have difficulty with social relations, yet are able to make great strides in their careers. Still others, unfortunately, remain unemployed, or work at jobs with low pay or low status. And many have difficulty sustaining relationships and family responsibilities.

And, of course, external demands also affect a person's ability to adapt and succeed. Challenges must be met as adults take on role changes and different levels of responsibility at work, or in school, or within the family. This might include taking on the responsibilities of being a parent while trying to maintain a full-time job or complete a college degree. Although all adults must deal with changing patterns of responsibility, those who have a learning disability may also have to tackle persistent academic difficulties, interpersonal problems, or a sense of helplessness or low self-esteem as a consequence of years of failure. Even those adults who are successful may still need to compensate for their disabilities and work harder to achieve their goals.

When we ask adults who have learning disabilities to identify the factors that have contributed most to their achievements, they point to an interaction of internal abilities and external supports like family, teachers, and mentors. The internal characteristics are all tied to self-determination, by which we mean an individual's ability and willingness to set goals and use strategies to control his or her life. To be self-determined, individuals must first accept the fact that they have a learning disability, evaluate their strengths and weaknesses, and then rely on their strengths to help them compensate for their weaknesses. Also, they must accept responsibility for both accomplishments and setbacks. Specialists who work with learning disabilities and related professionals in high schools, colleges, and even in the early grades are now teaching students self-advocacy and other strategies designed to promote understanding and self-determination. In the years to come, we hope to see ever-increasing numbers of young people exiting high school as self-determined adults.

Although it is clear that adults who have learning disabilities face many obstacles as they negotiate the demands of daily life, we have good reason to be optimistic. The numbers of young people with learning disabilities who are receiving high school diplomas and attending colleges and graduate schools are growing every day. Not suprisingly, students with learning disabilities who earn a high school diploma are more likely to be successful on the job than those who do not graduate. And those who continue to postsecondary school tend to get jobs more easily and advance in their careers to a greater degree than those with only a high school diploma.

Approximately 3 to 10 percent of the adult population has a learning disability. Some were diagnosed as children, but others struggled through school never knowing exactly why. They may have been labeled lazy or dumb or slow, despite high intelligence and strong motivation. Without diagnosis and help, they were filled with anger, fear, frustration, and self-doubt.

The children who were highlighted in articles and books when the field of learning disabilities was first emerging in the 1960s are now adults. The children for whom the special education law was first passed in 1975 are now adults. And all the children who had trouble in the 1950s, 1960s, and 1970s learning to read, write, and do mathematics (even though they were intelligent and were regularly attending school) are now adults. The field of learning disabilities, once almost exclusively involved in the education of children and adolescents, is now concerned with the needs of adults as well.

What we are finding out is that learning disabilities are expressed differently at different ages and stages of life. The impact of the disability on an adult is influenced by changing educational, social, personal, and occupational demands. Adults with learning disabilities cannot be regarded as children with learning disabilities grown up. Instead, adults with learning disabilities are a distinct group with unique characteristics and needs.

In recent years there has been an increased response to the growing number of adults who have learning disabilities. There are now legal mandates such as the Americans with Disabilities Act and programs in colleges, in communities, and in the workplace designed to address the varied needs of this population. Take, for example, the workplace. Employers are more than ever providing workplace support and accommodations. With accommodations, adults who have learning disabilities are more apt to stay in their jobs, perform in a productive manner, advance professionally, and, overall, feel self-satisfaction.

Employers want their workers to be proficient in reading, writing, and mathematical skills and to be able to apply these skills to solve problems. They expect employees to have good interpersonal skills, and be able to use technology and information systems. More and more educators and related professionals are recognizing these on-the-job demands, and through such initiatives as transition planning and programming are preparing young people, beginning at an early age, with the skills and competencies needed for the workplace. Career awareness is now being introduced in elementary-school classrooms, and such services as vocational counseling, job placement, and job coaching are offered in high schools throughout the country. Individual tutoring and small group instruction in basic skills, learning strategies, and specific subject matter are being provided to children who have learning disabilities at very young ages and continuing throughout their school years. And a range of support and intervention programs is now available for adults as well.

## OVERVIEW OF THE BOOK

There has been significant progress in the field of learning disabilities. We now know more about the course and nature of learning disabilities, and theories about learning are helping us develop better assessment measures and interventions, particularly for the adult. But to be effective, this ever-expanding knowledge base must be made available to both adults who have learning disabilities and the professionals who work with them. This book brings together the relevant and up-to-date information you will need if you are an adult with a learning disability, or have a child with one. We hope to provide readers with an understanding of their condition and offer practical ways to compensate.

We also believe that, in addition to readers with disabilities, professionals will be interested in both the theory and practical information that are included here.

The book covers:

• Definition, characteristics, and causes of a learning disability
• The assessment process

- Attention-deficit/ hyperactivity disorder
- Related psychosocial problems
- Impact of a learning disability on college and employment
- Vocational rehabilitation
- Types of intervention
- Legislation and legal cases

Chapters 1 and 2 provide an introduction and overview of learning disabilities and commonly used definitions in the field.

Chapter 3 turns to suggested causes or etiology of a learning disability. We know, for example, that the central nervous system controls learning, but significant advances in technology and research have helped pinpoint specific structures and functions of the brain that are associated with learning disabilities. Research also continues to support the fact that learning disabilities run in families.

Chapter 4 describes our cognitive or thinking systems—often called information processing and metacognitive systems. These systems provide us with an understanding of how we learn and the role each of us plays in making this happen. The information processing system has been likened to a computer because, like a computer, it receives, processes, and organizes information and stores it in memory. The metacognitive system has an executive function that allows us to control how we organize and retrieve information when necessary.

Chapter 5 provides a detailed description of the assessment process. For example, we describe the different settings and approaches, and give examples of some of the tests used to diagnose a learning disability. Getting tested as an adult may be a difficult step. But we believe that knowing what to expect, and understanding how testing will help, will make it easier.

Chapter 6 explains dyslexia, which is often discussed but little understood. Over the years, we have all probably read more on dyslexia than any other type of learning disability. But what is dyslexia and how do you know whether you have this disability? In order to answer questions like these, we define dyslexia and discuss some possible causes, as well as research findings and a clinical example of dyslexia in the adult.

A learning disability affects academic performance at all levels, and chapter 7 carefully reviews reading, writing, and mathematical problems.

Do all reading problems look alike? Does a writing problem necessarily mean poor handwriting? The answers will be found in this chapter.

Chapter 8 provides a detailed review of attention-deficit/hyperactivity disorder (ADHD) and its relationship to learning disabilities. Current statistics indicate that approximately 30 to 50 percent of children with a formally diagnosed learning disability have ADHD, and individuals with ADHD are also at risk for learning disabilities—probably as many as 10 to 25 percent. Since ADHD affects 3 to 5 percent of the adult population, many readers will want to know more about both disorders. The chapter provides the definition and what we know about the cause, the symptoms, and treatment approaches.

Chapter 9 describes psychosocial problems. While these are not the primary cause of a learning disability, they are associated with and contribute to problems in learning. For example, low self-esteem and passivity affect performance in the classroom and the workplace. The chapter will define and explain the different problems, and provide a review of some of the current theories and treatment approaches.

Chapter 10 reviews the different types of instructional approaches in use. We know that instruction in the development of cognitive strategies and academic skills is effective in improving performance across tasks and improving performance in both academic and work settings. We have seen how these interventions work.

The transition to college and employment is a significant turning point for any adult. Understanding how a learning disability can have an impact on performance in college and the workplace is essential in planning for these important steps. Chapters 11 and 12 provide the reader with information regarding transition issues, accommodations, and program models.

Chapter 13 reviews vocational rehabilitation services, which provide services to help individuals determine career goals and objectives.

In Chapter 14, we provide case studies and interviews with adults who have learning disabilities to highlight the fact that there are a range of learning problems and a range of individuals who have taken different and varied routes to success. You may have heard it said that Albert Einstein had a learning disability, but you will surely profit more from examples that are closer to home.

In chapter 15, we discuss the current directions in the field. Today the field of learning disabilities is working to help individuals become proactive and empowered. One must develop the skills and strategies needed to take control of and determine life's choices and directions. Success for adults who have learning disabilities is more likely than ever before, in part because of the increase in research and legal protection and the broad range of services and interventions now available.

Over the years, both federal and state laws have mandated services and protection for individuals with learning disabilities. Appendix A summarizes the relevant legislation and legal cases.

Turn to the Glossary at the end of the book for an explanation of terms.

# 2

# *What Is a Learning Disability?*

*I went through school struggling with reading and writing, believing that I was not "smart." It was not until I was an adult that I understood why I was having these problems. Learning that I could continue school and work toward my goals made such a difference to me—it changed my life.*

Sara had worked as a registered nurse in a large city hospital for over 10 years. While she held a responsible position and was considered good at what she did, she struggled with persistent learning problems. She reversed numbers and letters when reading. The content of her writing was not well organized. Her poor reading comprehension interfered, to some degree, with her job and her ability to read for pleasure. Fear of making an error made her overly anxious at work.

As a student, Sara had had difficulty with reading, spelling, and writing. In nursing school, she enlisted friends to read to her, but still she needed to spend more time than they did completing assignments and studying for exams. Sara always attributed these problems to the fact that she was not "smart." But, at thirty-five, she was less willing to accept this explanation. She wanted to continue her education and look for advancement at work. She was determined to see what help was available.

Sara's need to look for answers as an adult is not unusual. Five million to eleven million adults struggle with learning disabilities that affect their reading and writing skills or their ability to calculate numbers or to reason mathematically. Their struggles continue way beyond childhood because they never mastered certain basic skills or learned how to rely on strategies that could help them overcome their problems. In some cases, they never developed the social skills we all need to navigate in the world. We now know that learning disabilities persist throughout one's life, and can affect performance in college and on the job.

## WHAT DOES A LEARNING DISABILITY LOOK LIKE?

Sara's lifelong difficulty with reading and writing had nothing to do with not being "smart." Most individuals who have a learning disability are of average to above average intelligence and therefore have the intellectual potential to succeed at school and in careers. But they often do not reach this potential. While effort and motivation are important for success, it is clearly unfair to say of someone with a learning disability that he or she "just needs to try harder." No matter how hard Sara worked, her problems did not go away.

We know that a learning disability is caused by specific dysfunction within the central nervous system. The central nervous system, made up of the brain and the spinal cord, controls everything we do: our ability to process and think about language and to express ourselves verbally, as well as our ability to process nonverbal information, including art or music.

Sara's symptoms included reversing or rotating numbers (*6* for *9*), letters (*b* for *d*; *p* for *q*), and words (*was* for *saw*; *on* for *no*) when writing; omitting letters and sounds; and making sound and word substitutions when reading (*tril* for *trial*; *then* for *there*). Such problems make it difficult to decode words, and these decoding errors are most evident when reading aloud.

Though never diagnosed, Sara's symptoms became evident in first grade, when formal reading instruction began. As we learn to read we must of course master the alphabet, which is like a code, and learn the relationship between letters and sounds. Reading is a process of decoding the clusters of letters, converting them into words, and then attaching meaning to the words.

In many cases, problems with *phonological processing*—the ability to receive, transform, remember, and retrieve the sounds of oral language—interfere with the acquisition of reading skills. Phonological processing involves the ability to separate a word into its component parts or blend sounds to construct a word. Problems with these skills make it very hard for the beginning reader to achieve fluency.

Comprehension of written material depends on accurate and fluent decoding, a good vocabulary, and comprehension of the grammatical structure of sentences. When these skills are not developed—that is, when they are slow and labored—the reader must devote more energy and effort to identifying and comprehending each individual word, rather than constructing meaning from an entire paragraph or from general context.

For many years, researchers believed that the reader automatically moved from reading the words on a page to comprehending, without participating in the process of constructing meaning. But recent research points to the fact that the reader plays an active role: using background knowledge about the subject, calling on appropriate strategies for both decoding and comprehension, and applying the right amount of attention and concentration. Reading strategies are now considered essential components of the reading process. These might include paraphrasing while reading or summarizing afterward to help with comprehension. Competent readers are able to evaluate the reading task and select strategies that are a "good fit" or match to the task.

In Sara's case, she read slowly and had to reread material several times, so she found it difficult to comprehend content or recall important facts when questioned about them later. Unlike good readers, she did not rely on strategies that could help her. She also struggled with writing. Many times she was ashamed to submit patient reports because she knew they were filled with spelling, punctuation, and grammatical errors and were not organized or structured well. Her reports never reflected her knowledge or keen insight into patient care.

Writing problems can be seen at any age, although they become more evident as academic or work demands increase. While Sara knew what she wanted to say, she had trouble getting started, focusing on the essential facts, and editing effectively. She tended to use the same words over and over. This was so different from her spoken language, which was rich and varied. Not surprisingly, it took her a long time and a good deal of effort to complete her reports.

Her mathematical skills, though, were more than adequate. But there are people with learning disabilities who have problems understanding mathematical concepts or difficulty solving verbal or written mathematical problems. These problems may stem from more than one source, including inadequate spatial or directional sense and difficulty understanding abstract symbols or the language of mathematics. To use a basic example, someone who does not have a good understanding of concepts such as "plus" and "minus" is going to find it hard to identify the process needed to solve a mathematical problem. Learning strategies will be of great help to this person.

Sara was also troubled by her erratic performance at work. Some days, she would be fine. But when she was fatigued or stressed, she found her attention was poor and she made more than the usual number of errors. At these times, she did not feel in control and usually needed to take a break and call on the support of friends to help her get back on track.

While Sara felt her social life to be a strength, some individuals who have learning disabilities have difficulty in social situations because they cannot perceive others' needs and make or keep friends. Relationships with family and friends and associates on the job may suffer. As a way of compensating, an individual may avoid social situations altogether and thus become isolated. Others may struggle with low self-esteem and a lack of assertiveness, which can lead to self-fulfilling prophecies of failure. Moreover, repeated negative experiences in school and at home can discourage an individual from even trying.

Many individuals who have learning disabilities have difficulty planning ahead and then evaluating their performance in academic courses or work-related tasks. Planning involves the ability to determine the outlines of a task and the skills it will require. Planning helps us generate strategies or know when to ask for outside help. We are not always conscious of initiating this type of planning because so many tasks are performed automatically, such as remembering a frequently called phone number by using a mnemonic, or writing notes in a book or on a memo. But when tasks are new or complex, active planning is needed.

Other learning problems may stem from an inability to manage one's time effectively to get something done on schedule. For example, many college students do not leave sufficient time to research and write a term paper, and end up frantically completing it the night before it is due. Or a manager may delay writing a budget or marketing report, finding it hard to begin.

In order to use strategies at school, at home, or on the job, we need to be aware of ourselves as learners. Researchers have suggested that each of us has our own built-in executive function that directs and controls our actions. If this "executive" is efficient and aware of individual skills and the strategies needed to accomplish a task, the appropriate plan of action can be put into effect. If the plan is unsuccessful, then the executive reevaluates and initiates a new course of action. Individuals who have learning disabilities have a less efficient executive, the theory goes, and are therefore less able to generate and use effective strategies in their personal and professional lives.

In addition to learning disabilities, a large number of adults suffer from attention-deficit/hyperactivity disorder (ADHD). ADHD affects an individual's ability to focus and concentrate on school or work tasks, and to make good use of strategies. The struggle to achieve is so much harder with the added burden of ADHD.

Although external factors do not cause a learning disability, we know that they do play a significant role in learning. It is well documented that the environment we live and work in influences and helps to shape our learning patterns, behavior, and sense of self. Research has consistently shown that the type and quality of support provided both at school and within the home are strong determinants of success in school, at work, or in one's personal life. For example, a supportive family, early identification of learning problems, and appropriate intervention may make all the difference in helping an individual compensate for the disability.

Learning disabilities are found throughout the world and in all socioeconomic groups—they are not bound by culture or language. Approximately the same number of males as females have learning disabilities, and the problem tends to run in families. Many prominent figures in politics, science, and the arts are reported to have had a learning disability, among them Nelson Rockefeller, Winston Churchill, Albert Einstein, Thomas Edison, and Auguste Rodin. Einstein, for example, was described as having difficulty learning a foreign language and mathematics—of all things! He also struggled with other academic subjects and with writing.

Is Sara's case typical? Yes. Also typical of adults thirty-five years or older is the fact that she and her family had little or no understanding of her disability throughout her childhood and adolescence. Since Sara received inadequate support while in school, she did not learn to use coping strategies. The field of learning disabilities was just developing in the 1960s, and special education services were limited until legislation provided the impetus, framework, and funding for care. Sara did not benefit from the support of these services because her teachers did not adequately identify her needs and because her parents were not educated about the nature of her disability or the rights Sara had to a quality education. Sara was lucky. She had enough intelligence and ability to compensate. She managed to get by, though she never worked up to her potential. Her teachers just thought she lacked motivation. It was not until she looked for help as an adult that the cause of her intense struggle became clear.

## DEFINING A LEARNING DISABILITY

As we have already said, a learning disability is an umbrella term that includes different subsets of problems. But what exactly does this mean? It may mean difficulty with reading decoding, reading comprehension, written expression, mathematical calculations or reasoning, and oral language, or a combination of these. While a number of definitions have been formulated and used over the years, each has its shortcomings. The definitions most often used talk about a significant difference between ability and achievement in one or more areas, such as reading, written expression, or mathematics. These definitions exclude other disabilities such as sensory impairment, mental retardation, social and emotional disturbance, or environmental influence as the primary cause of learning problems. Some definitions also note that a learning disability is caused by central nervous system dysfunction.

### Two Widely Used Definitions

The two definitions that will be be discussed are widely used. One is the definition incorporated into federal law, and the other was developed by the Interagency Committee on Learning Disabilities.

#### *The Individuals with Disabilities Education Act (IDEA)*

The definition in the Individuals with Disabilities Education Act (IDEA) is the most commonly used in the field of education. It first appeared in the initial version of the law in 1975 and then in the reauthorization in 1990, as well as in its most recent reauthorization in 1997. This definition guides educational practice and has two parts, the first of which reads:

> The term "specific learning disability" means those children who have a disorder in one or more of the basic psychological processes involved in understanding or in using language, spoken or written, which disorder may manifest itself in imperfect ability to listen, think, speak, read, write, spell, or do mathematical calculations. The term includes such conditions as perceptual handicaps, brain injury, minimal brain dysfunction, dyslexia, and developmental aphasia. The term does not include a learning problem which is primarily the result of visual, hearing, or motor handicaps, of mental retardation, of emotional disturbance, or of environmental, cultural, or economic disadvantage.

Notice that this definition uses the term "basic psychological processes." This term is not in common use today. When used, it refers to cognitive abilities presumed to underlie learning, like memory, auditory perception, visual perception, spoken language, and thinking.

The second part of the definition sets the guidelines for classification for school-aged children in the public schools. It states that a student is considered to have a learning disability if he or she does not achieve at levels commensurate with his age or ability, when afforded appropriate instructional experiences—in other words, when there is a significant discrepancy between ability and achievement in one or more of seven areas. These areas are oral expression, listening comprehension, written expression, basic reading, reading comprehension, mathematical calculation, and reasoning.

### *National Joint Committee on Learning Disabilities (NJCLD)*

The National Joint Committee on Learning Disabilities (NJCLD), an organization of representatives from various professional groups involved with learning disabilities, formulated the following definition in 1994:

> Learning Disabilities is a general term that refers to a heterogeneous group of disorders manifested by significant difficulties in the acquisition of listening, speaking, reading, writing, reasoning, or mathematical abilities.

These disorders are intrinsic to the individual and presumed to be due to central nervous system dysfunction. Problems in self-regulatory behaviors, perception, and social interaction may exist with learning disabilities, but do not by themselves constitute a learning disability. Even though a learning disability may occur concomitantly with other handicapping conditions (for example, sensory impairment, mental retardation, social and emotional disturbance) or environmental influences (such as cultural differences, insufficient or inappropriate instruction, psychogenic factors), it is not a result of those conditions or influences.

There are differences between the federal and the NJCLD definitions, which are outlined below:

### NJCLD Definition
1. Does not mention psychological processes.
2. Notes that the learning disabled population is heterogeneous.
3. Notes that learning problems are related to factors within the individual, and not to the environment or educational system.
4. Notes that central nervous system dysfunction—that is, a disorder in the structure or function of the brain—underlies problems in learning.
5. Does not include an exclusionary clause, but states that a person can have a learning disability along with one or more of these other conditions.
6. Adds self regulatory and social difficulties to other problems in learning such as speaking, listening, and reading. However, a person cannot be said to have a learning disability on the basis of self-regulatory or social problems alone.

### Federal Definition
1. Notes that learning disabilities are due to a disorder in basic psychological processes.
2. Does not include the fact that learning disorders are intrinsic to the individual or due to central nervous system dysfunction.
3. Includes an exclusionary clause, ruling out factors such as sensory or motor impairments and emotional disturbance.
4. Does not mention self-regulatory or social problems.

## Other Definitions

### *The Diagnostic and Statistical Manual of Mental Disorders, Fourth Edition*

*The Diagnostic and Statistical Manual of Mental Disorders, Fourth Edition* (American Psychiatric Association, 1994), referred to as DSM-IV, is the classification system used by mental health professionals for disorders of children and adults. The first version of DSM was published in 1952. In 1980, DSM-III provided a comprehensive classification of childhood and developmental disorders. DSM-III-R, published in 1987, and DSM-IV, published in 1994, use similar criteria. DSM-IV classifies learning disorders as a disorder of childhood. There are no distinct criteria for diagnosing this condition in adults.

Learning disabilities are defined according to the following disorders: reading disorder, mathematics disorder, disorder of written expression, and learning disorder "not otherwise specified"—which means they have the characteristics of learning disorders but do not satisfy the full criteria for the above categories. Like IDEA, emphasis is on academic underachievement, using a discrepancy-based formula.

### *Statutory Definitions*

Statutory definitions are those that have become part of federal, state, or local laws, for example, those included in IDEA, Section 504 of the Rehabilitation Act, and the Americans with Disabilities Act (ADA). Section 504 and ADA both use the following *functional* definition of a disability. This refers to *all* types of disabilities, including learning disabilities. A person is considered to be handicapped or have a disability if he or she "has a physical or mental impairment that substantially limits one or more major activities, has a record or history of such an impairment, or is regarded as having such an impairment."

While specific learning disabilities fall under the definition of "mental impairment," neither a learning disability nor attention-deficit/hyperactivity disorder is mentioned in the ADA or in its employment regulations.

### *Federal and State Agency Definitions*

Most federal and state agencies have depended on more than one definition. Many have relied on Public Law 94-142 and its revision, IDEA, although these definitions are not specific to the adult population. However, the Rehabilitation Services Administration (RSA) developed a definition to identify adults with learning disabilities.

Before 1981, the Rehabilitation Services Administration (RSA) recognized only the classification of mental and physical disabilities. Learning disabilities were viewed as educational problems, which did not fall under these categories. In 1981, the RSA issued a policy directive, making a specific learning disability a medically recognized disability, and, in 1985, it was classified as a neuropsychological condition. The definition states:

> Individuals who have a disorder due to central nervous system dysfunction involving perceiving, understanding and/or using concepts through verbal (spoken or written language) or non-verbal means. This disorder manifests itself with difficulties in one or more of the following areas: attention, reasoning, memory, communicating, reading, writing, spelling, calculation, coordination, social competence and emotional maturity. These disorders may constitute, in an adult, an employment handicap. The condition has an impact on employment.

The RSA definition suggests that a learning disability is a lifelong condition due to central nervous system dysfunction, and highlights problems with attention, memory, coordination, social competence, and emotional maturity. These areas are relevant in considering eligibility for vocational placement. The definition does not specify the use of discrepancy criteria.

# 3

# *What Causes a Learning Disability?*

*When I found out I had a learning disability, I was
relieved. I had known that my father had dyslexia that
went untreated. I came to realize that having a learning
disability was all right. It meant I wasn't stupid.*

A learning disability is often misunderstood. We have frequently been
asked: What is the cause of a learning disability? Is it biological or due to
the environment? Is it inherited?

We know that a learning disability is biological. During one's life,
environmental factors such as schooling and personal supports can certainly make learning easier or more difficult, but the evidence shows that
those who have a learning disability exhibit a subtle difference in the
structure and function of their central nervous systems. This difference
affects the cognitive processes that are essential to learning.

## THE ROLE OF THE CENTRAL NERVOUS SYSTEM

The complex and intricate communications network known as the central
nervous system regulates and coordinates everything we do, including
learning. The central nervous system includes the brain and the spinal
cord. The spinal cord relays messages, via nerve cells, between the brain
and other parts of the body.

Learning is a function of the brain. The brain stem, the cerebellum, and
the cerebrum are the key components of the brain (see Figure 1). The
largest area of the brain is the cerebrum (located at the top of the brain),
and it is here that higher thought processes such as memory, reasoning,
and learning are centered. A large groove, or fissure, divides the cerebrum
into two halves or hemispheres, the right and the left. While the two hemispheres are almost identical in structure, they differ in function. Struc-

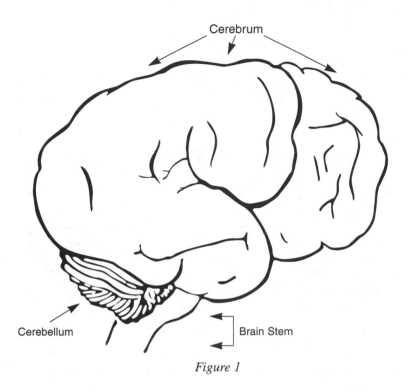

*Figure 1*

turally, both hemispheres have a strip of cells that control motor activity as well as four regions called lobes (frontal lobe, temporal lobe, occipital lobe, and parietal lobe), divided from one another by fissures. The strip of motor cells in one hemisphere controls the movements of the opposite side of the body. For example, the action of the right foot and hand originates in the left side of the brain, the action of the left foot and hand in the right side. A lobe in one hemisphere communicates with its counterpart in the other hemisphere through a bundle of nerve fibers in the center called the corpus callosum. (See Figure 2 for a diagram of the structure of the brain.)

The left hemisphere controls most language processing, as well as logic and organization, although information does flow between hemispheres. Each hemisphere has its own responsibilities, but for most learning tasks the two hemispheres work together. Complex activities require the coordination of several regions within both hemispheres, each activated to a different degree. The right hemisphere is concerned primarily with nonverbal stimuli and directs such abilities as spatial perception,

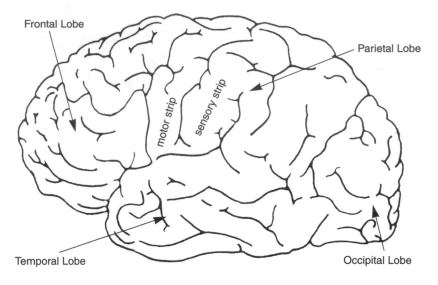

*Figure 2*

visual imagery, directional orientation, sequencing of time, and appreciation of art and music.

The brain is composed of 180 billion cells, 80 billion of which are directly involved in the processing of information. Each nerve cell has a cell body, numerous projections called dendrites that conduct impulses to the cell body, and an axon that directs impulses away from the cell body. Dendrites and axons of neighboring cells communicate with one another via chemical agents called neurotransmitters.

If a particular brain region is not functioning effectively, a person's ability to perform the tasks normally assumed by that area is diminished. The brain has billions of nerve cells, though, and sometimes cells from one region can, to varying degrees, take over the jobs of another. We refer to this phenomenon as the *plasticity* of the brain. The degree to which a person can recover from brain trauma is dependent, in part, on the person's age, the location and size of the damage, and the type and extent of rehabilitation or retraining the person receives. Despite the plasticity of the brain, complete recovery after brain trauma is the exception rather than the rule. For some behaviors there may be no recovery at all.

## THE BRAIN AND LEARNING: A HISTORICAL VIEW

The field of learning disabilities has its historical roots in the work of physicians, psychologists, and educators who linked brain abnormalities to problems with language and language-based abilities such as reading and writing, as well as with a person's difficulty with perception, organization, and attention.

The term *learning disability* was first introduced to the field of special education in 1963 by Samuel Kirk, an educator, speaking at a conference for concerned parents and professionals. Dr. Kirk was looking to develop services for children of normal intelligence who were having significant difficulty learning and performing in school but who did not fit into existing disability categories like mental retardation, emotional disturbance, and sensory impairment. These children exhibited uneven patterns of development and had unique strengths and weaknesses in a range of academic and behavioral areas.

More than one hundred years before Kirk's talk, the literature described characteristics we now associate with the term learning disability and attributed these characteristics to brain dysfunction. As early as the 1800s, physicians, using autopsies of adults who had suffered from stroke, accident, or disease, discovered that damage to a part of the brain would result in the loss of the ability to speak. Somewhat later, connections were made between brain function and reading and writing, connections based on clinical impressions from work with children.

For example, James Hinshelwood, a physician, worked with children who had normal vision, motivation, and intelligence, but were unable to interpret written language. He termed their condition *congenital word blindness* and suggested that the problem was related to a specific difference in the structure of the brain. Samuel T. Orton, a neurologist, proposed that the lack of dominance of the left hemisphere, the predominant site of language, accounted for reading disabilities in children. Like Hinshelwood, Orton worked with children who had significant difficulty acquiring reading skills and whose reading and writing was marked by errors such as reversals of letters and words. He termed this condition *strephosymbolia*, meaning "twisted symbols." The constellation of characteristics both Hinshelwood and Orton identified is today associated with the learning disorder dyslexia.

As one group of clinicians, like Hinshelwood and Orton, was associating brain dysfunction with reading and writing, another linked the brain dysfunction with certain behavioral symptoms. Kurt Goldstein, a physician treating World War I veterans, found that soldiers who had suffered head injuries showed perceptual impairments, distractibility and perseveration (being locked into producing the same action again, and again), symptoms that persisted even after recuperation.

By the middle of the twentieth century, Alfred Strauss, a neuropsychiatrist, and Heinz Werner, a psychologist, were using information gained from research on the brain to better understand, assess, and teach children who exhibited characteristics such as excessive motor activity, poor organizational abilities, distractibility, perceptual difficulties, awkwardness with motor tasks, and perseveration—behaviors strikingly similar to those of Goldstein's soldiers. They speculated that the learning characteristics and behaviors these children exhibited were due to some form of brain injury sustained within the birth process. While some children did indeed have brain injury, for many, however, brain dysfunction was assumed on the basis of these clinical symptoms.

## UPDATE ON RESEARCH

Initially much of our information about the brain was based on postmortem anatomical studies of brain sections. In the late 1970s and 80s, neuroscientists, most notably Norman Geschwind and Albert Galabruda, studied the brains of deceased individuals who were reported to have been dyslexic and found anomalies in language and language-related areas. More recently, advanced technologies have allowed scientists to study the working, living brain. Results of these studies have lent support to the autopsy findings. For example, research with magnetic resonance imaging (MRI), the neuroimaging device that transforms signals derived from magnetic fields into an anatomical image on a video screen, shows that the frontal region of the brain of children with dyslexia is different than it is in those without this disability. Similarly, work with brain electrical activity mapping (BEAM), which uses computers to map electrical brain waves, reveals that the electrical activity in the language-related areas of the brain of individuals who have dyslexia is different from those who do not have dyslexia. While the majority of research has focused on children, some recent work has been done with adults. In 1991, for example, Karen Gross-Glen and colleagues, using positron emission tomography (PET), which measures the metabolic activity of the brain, observed twenty-five adults with dyslexia as they performed reading tasks, and found significant differences in frontal and occipital areas of the brain.

Information about this work has been reported in the media, so it is not surprising that many people who suspect they may have a learning disability ask their doctors if this technology can be used to diagnose their problems. But these techniques are being used for research only, not yet to diagnose an individual learning disability.

Diagnosis of a learning disability relies on an assessment that uses a battery of achievement and cognitive tests to determine whether a significant discrepancy exists between ability and achievement. Given that technology is not yet available for clinical use, we have no hard-and-fast evidence of a central nervous system dysfunction.

## WHAT CAUSES THE SUBTLE BRAIN DYSFUNCTION?

We have a number of possible explanations to help us understand why there are differences in the structure and function of the brain in individuals who have learning disabilities, but there is still much to learn. Prior to birth, during the birth process, or directly after birth, there may be some trauma to the brain, perhaps because of an inadequate supply of oxygen, nutrients, or blood flow. Or, perhaps, during the course of fetal development there is irregular development of the brain. We also know that the mother's use of alcohol or drugs during pregnancy may play a part. A genetic predisposition may also be a factor. And some individuals may have an imbalance in the neurochemistry of the brain. Research suggests a link between levels of neurotransmitters and problems with attention and impulsivity.

### The Role of Heredity

Most likely, Sara had a genetic predisposition to a learning disability. Her father has a learning disability, as does her brother, uncle, and daughter.

Numerous studies conducted within the past thirty years, often in the form of family and twin studies, indicate that there is a 35 to 45 percent chance of inheriting a learning disability. Over the years, researchers have looked to identify a possible gene or genes that might be associated with a learning disability, but none has been isolated as yet. It is likely that more than a single gene accounts for the full spectrum of this condition, considering the heterogeneity of the population that has learning disabilities.

## EXTRINSIC FACTORS

As previously mentioned, extrinsic factors such as instruction, school curriculum, and home environment influence learning, but such variables do not cause a learning disability. The effect of the environment has been well documented in early intervention studies. We know, for example, that providing special education services to children younger than five years old who show developmental delays is crucial to support their capacity to learn. Beginning intervention when a child is older significantly reduces the ability to modify and encourage growth. In fact, we have a great deal of evidence that early intervention can accelerate cognitive and social growth and prevent subsequent behavioral problems. We spoke earlier of the plasticity of the brain. The younger the child, the more plastic the brain.

Intervention at a young age can also help the family, empowering parents to be an essential part of their children's learning and ultimately improving interactions between children and parents. With early intervention, some presenting symptoms can be overcome, others perhaps ameliorated, and secondary difficulties that can compound the disability, such as psychosocial problems, can be avoided. When Sara was very young, few, if any, early childhood special education programs existed in her community, particularly for children with only mild disabilities. Now special education programs for young children are mandated by law.

The school environment plays a critical role in learning. This includes the tasks we require individuals to perform, the learning setting we create, and the support we do or do not provide. These factors can greatly affect functioning at all ages and influence both short-term and ultimate success. Successful adults with learning disabilities have stressed to us the importance of these instructional factors. They have reported that small class size, availability of individualized tutoring, and teachers' willingness and ability to use a range of instructional techniques to accommodate diverse learning styles eased some of their learning difficulties and contributed to their achievements in later life. They knew they needed to work harder, and they benefited from teachers who used innovative approaches.

Interactions at home, school, or work also affect self-perception and self-esteem, which in turn can influence learning. Research tells us that children and adolescents who have a learning disability tend more often to be rejected by both their teachers and peers than their classmates without the disability. Certainly such rejection would contribute to problems with self-esteem. In addition, a history of repeated academic failure may leave them with a sense of incompetence, low motivation, and unfavorable attitudes toward learning and school. Throughout their lives, individuals who have a learning disability may never know the satisfaction that comes from recognition, achievement, and affection. On the other hand, strong emotional support from family, friends, and teachers in the early years as well as in later life can help help them enormously in dealing with academic and social/emotional challenges.

We know that at each critical stage of development, there is a shifting balance between *risk factors*, or stressful events that make a person vulnerable, and *protective factors*, which make him or her resilient. In order for a person to adapt well, there needs to be a balance between these stressful events, such as academic hurdles and peer rejection, and protective factors, such as emotional support from parents, teachers, and friends. And, of course, a person's individual pattern of strengths and weaknesses is a critical variable.

While Sara did struggle, to varying degrees, throughout her school career, and there were times when she did indeed feel "stupid," the encouragement of her family, some teachers, and a few close friends helped her adapt and compensate. "School was hard," she says,

> often very hard, but I was lucky to have some very supportive teachers and, with my parents' help and lots of extra effort on my part and perseverance,

I managed to complete school and become a nurse. I learned to roll with the punches. I wish, though, I had known about my learning disability. I think that knowledge and the understanding of what a learning disability is might have made my growing-up years somewhat easier. I never knew why school was so much harder for me than it was for my friends.

# 4

## *How We Process Information*

*I always had significant memory problems. . . . If I was
told to do things, twelve seconds later, it was gone. . . . I
couldn't follow the steps to a task.*

From the time of Aristotle and Plato, philosophers and psychologists have
attempted to define and explain the elusive concept of memory. Aristotle
used the analogy of a wax tablet. He suggested that the size and quality of
the tablet determined an individual's success in learning and storing
information in memory.

In the late 1800s, William James proposed a spatial metaphor, the
house. In this analogy, specific memories are like objects in a house. It is
assumed that these objects are retrieved through a random search process.
James separated memory into two systems: *primary* memory, which is at
the unconscious level, and *secondary* memory, which is in conscious control. While these theories and ideas have changed considerably over the
years, the spatial and search metaphors are still applicable.

With the growth of technology in the 1950s and 1960s, particularly the
computer, advances were made in conceptualizing and understanding
how the human mind operates in the process of thinking, learning, and
remembering. The computer aptly demonstrates how information flows
through a system, in stages, moving from input or reception of information into storage or the memory system. It was suggested that similar
operations occurred in the working of the human mind.

## THE HUMAN MIND AS A COMPUTER

The computer analogy provides a dynamic framework to study how
humans process information. By *dynamic*, we mean that the individual
plays an active role in processing, storing, and retrieving all types of
information. This is done through the use of control functions, similar to

those on your computer, such as "search" and "save." For example, when searching for information, you initiate a set of activities, such as reviewing the directory or store of mental files, and then retrieve the file you need.

The information-processing system, as it has come to be called, is one of a number of ways of looking at the steps and activities we take from learning to recall. This approach is useful in helping us to understand how and under what conditions we take active control of these steps. It is also a significant shift from some of the early theories, which viewed learning as a passive activity in a system with a limited capacity. The information-processing system is well integrated into current research and practice in cognitive psychology and education.

## The Information-Processing System

Cognitive psychologists have used the information-processing system to help explain the different stages and processes involved in cognitive or intellectual functioning, or simply in thinking. When we talk about cognition or intelligence, we are referring to our ability to receive, transform, store, and use language and other types of information under a variety of conditions. Cognitive functioning or thinking involves a set of complex and discrete stages and skills that are needed to connect what we already know with the processing and organization of new information.

The information-processing system drawn from the computer analogy has been expanded by psychologists to include two essential components: the basic hardware or structure, including attention and the different memory centers, such as short- and long-term memory; and the executive system, including one's knowledge about the world, the proposed executive that controls the system, and the strategies needed to perform a range of tasks effectively.

This system provides us with a workable format that helps explain how individuals perform simple tasks as well as complex ones, such as comprehending what we read, solving mathematical computations, or recalling names or facts on demand. But why are some of us able to recall the details of a novel or movie, while others forget even major events? The information-processing system helps to explain some of these differences.

The system includes three memory centers: sensory register, short-term memory, and long-term memory.

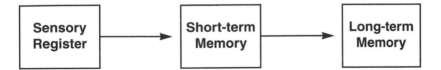

Like the computer, the human mind receives signals ("input"), performs processing functions such as thinking, decision making, and storage, and creates "output," such as writing, talking, or gesturing. At the initial stage, signals are received through the sense of vision, hearing, touch, taste, or smell. They reach the *sensory register*, where they are held briefly for rapid recognition. If preserved, the signals are sent to *short-term memory*, often referred to as working memory. This stage is also a temporary storage center, with about five to twenty seconds allotted for conscious attention and processing. We have this very brief amount of time to attend to, perceive, and think about the information, then either send it to *long-term memory* or "bump" it and displace it by new signals.

This is an efficient system. While we are all bombarded with a good deal of sensory information, we cannot process all this stimuli, nor is it all relevant to us. Taking a familiar route to school or to work, we may not notice the architectural features of the buildings around us. Mingling at a cocktail party, we may not pick up specific voices or conversations within the overall din. Yet, one morning, we notice the roof of one of these buildings, and immediately associate it with one seen the previous day. In this case, we have made the conscious decision to attend to and process the image of the roof at the perceptual level. Otherwise, it would be lost, never gaining access to the system. When we refer to the perceptual level, we mean the step beyond receiving information through the senses. Perception requires thinking. When we perceive something touched or seen, we are identifying and thinking about these signals in order to make rapid decisions whether to maintain and then store the information. When we tune into what seems to be an interesting conversation, we have decided to perceive and process the information. In the case of the roof, the perceived image and association will be stored.

A computer silently performs the operations needed, following an appropriate command, but what operations take place in the human mind when information moves through the different stages into storage? Here is where the executive system comes into play. The idea is that planning and strategies are needed to hold or maintain information in short-term memory until it is identified, processed, and then moved into long-term storage. Such strategies might include *rehearsal*, which is reviewing or repeating the material, or *grouping*, often referred to as *chunking*. For example, if you were asked to retain and repeat a series of numbers like 2, 4, 3, 5, 1, 2, you might benefit from chunking them as 24, 35, 12, which would be more efficient.

Long-term memory is a permanent memory store, which has an unlimited capacity and time frame. That is, we can save indeterminate amounts of information indefinitely. But, in order to retrieve information effectively, we must store it in a highly organized manner—like a filing system, where each cluster of information is identified and labeled. In this way, we can find the category and related facts when we need them.

## Schema

Each category, cluster, or file of information we store in long-term memory is called a *schema*. Schemas include both general and specific knowledge about a subject. When we learn something that is unfamiliar, a new schema is generated, as when we make up a new file folder at the office. If you are taking a course in biology for the first time, a hypothesized file is opened, labeled "Biology." Relevant information such as vocabulary and concepts can be added and stored in a format in this file. If you had studied biology before, then the existing file and schema can be retrieved and expanded, making learning the second time more efficient. Using schemas to organize and structure information is helpful in triggering recall and in making appropriate decisions when new information is received. It is certainly faster and more efficient to identify a specific file when it is needed than to search randomly through a cabinet with no labels.

Because long-term memory contains such a varied and vast store of information, it is suggested that this information is organized into two discrete memory centers: declarative and procedural. *Declarative memory* is a storage of facts and events, while *procedural memory* refers to memory for performing varying skills and strategies, such as the steps needed to ride a bicycle. Declarative memory has been further divided into two categories, episodic and semantic. *Episodic memory* includes temporal-spatial (time and space) experience and autobiographical events, while *semantic memory* is a "thesaurus" that includes language, symbols, rules, and generalizations. Clearly, there is a good deal of interaction between these memory centers, since most of the time we retrieve complex sets of information and procedures.

What we know about the world, our knowledge base, includes the content of these memory stores. The goal is to be able to access or retrieve this knowledge with ease. This appears to depend on how well the material is clustered and organized, as well as on our ability to utilize appropriate search strategies for retrieval. Research has shown that the more elaborate the schema, meaning the more rich and detailed the network of ideas and related facts, the better the recall. For example, after reading *Hamlet*, we might set up a schema that includes not only the events in the play, but a network of ideas consisting of the historical context of the play, the psychological implications of Hamlet's behavior, and our impressions after seeing a great stage production. These elaborations help us to understand the play, as well as to provide personally meaningful cues that are useful for retrieval. We have all had the experience of not being able to recall an acquaintance's name, or the facts we studied for an examination. These gaps or delays in retrieval may be due to the fact that the information was not well organized or associated, or that we used inappropriate strategies. For example, if you read *Hamlet* without fully understanding Shakespeare's language or the character's actions, then you would develop a limited schema. You may be able to retrieve the file, but it may be lacking in interpretative information or facts. Or the file may not be found at all. There are times when we read "passively," especially when we are tired, and find that we have understood and retained little of the content. Clearly, at these times, minimal processing and analysis are being done, and the information is not being properly stored for later use.

While we need conscious and active processing and strategies, our personal experience, knowledge, and views of the world also guide us in transforming and organizing all levels and types of information. In other words, who we are, what we know, how we think about things, our experiences, and what is meaningful to us serve as guidelines and organizing frameworks. This helps to explain why people may have different interpretations for the same movie or novel. Each of us restructures and reorganizes learning and experience along very personal dimensions.

## Metamemory and Metacognition

The term *metamemory* was first used in 1970 by John Flavell, a developmental psychologist. It refers to our knowledge about our own memory abilities—that is, knowing what makes it easy or hard to remember things and what types of information we remember best. We also use the term *metacognition* to refer to an awareness of what we know, how we learn best, and how we apply this knowledge when using strategies. "Meta" skills, then, include what we know ("declarative knowledge") and what we do ("procedural knowledge"). These are similar to the categories noted under long-term memory. The concepts of metamemory and metacognition are used to explain and describe how individuals use insight and knowledge in making conscious decisions regarding strategy use. The emphasis on conscious control suggests a complex set of responsibilities for the individual and raises the question, How do we manage to accomplish this effectively?

## The Executive Function

A number of researchers in psychology suggest that we have what is referred to as an *executive*, which serves as an internal manager, directing and controlling our use of strategies. The executive has become an essential feature of information-processing and "meta theories." Given the overwhelming amount of information we must process and the skills we must engage in each day, the notion of some kind of internal executive makes sense. In fact, this notion may help us to understand why some of us may forget to write down important phone numbers, while others use efficient strategies to deal with the many problems at home or at work.

The executive uses what we know about ourselves to direct essential cognitive activities. These include learning new information, storing and retrieving facts, and performing tasks effectively and efficiently. This responsibility involves complex planning. Planning means that we use what we know in selecting the best strategies to accomplish a task. To plan effectively for a sales meeting, we might generate appropriate statistics or budget figures or coordinate the sequence of presentations with other members of the team. At school, planning involves reviewing course material to determine what is hard or easy and deciding what operations can be used to solve problems, or what facts must be stored.

The executive also has ongoing responsibility—checking, monitoring, and evaluating results by asking the following questions: Is the approach or strategy working? Was the sales meeting a success? The actions of the executive are directed toward a specific goal, in the same way that an executive would perform within a high-powered organization, where anticipated results and outcomes are evaluated and documented. In order to operate effectively, the executive must have access to meta knowledge and a range of strategies. If a plan does not work, the executive evaluates what went wrong and why. This information is then put to use the next time, so that the same mistakes are not repeated.

We do know that the executive is not always called upon for action. For example, our own address and phone number are so familiar that we can retrieve these numbers automatically, without a conscious plan. In this case we say that metamemory is "bypassed." However, when we are faced with new or complex tasks, the executive must be activated, identify what is needed, and evaluate and implement the best plan of action.

## Development of Meta Skills

Metacognition and metamemory are part of our cognitive framework, and as such are thought to follow a similar developmental line. By and large the young child formulates and expresses concepts and ideas along concrete dimensions that can be seen or touched. This tie to the external world is coupled with a lack of metacognitive insight. In other words, the young child is less conscious of what he can do and less able to evaluate and use strategies independently. For example, if a kindergartener was asked if she could remember a long list of names, she might suggest that she could, with a good deal of bravado. But, when tested, she recalls few of them. With development, however, there is a gradual change in conceptual thinking and the "bag of tricks" children use.

From the late elementary years through adolescence and even into adulthood, we continue to learn to think in abstract terms, use abstract concepts, and engage in self-analysis. The development of insight, along with experience, helps us target and use appropriate strategies that match the tasks to be done. There are also changes in contextual demands that require us to learn new strategies. For example, there are general strategies that we all use, such as organizing our day. But we must also develop specialized strategies for school that help us learn the names of the bones of the hand or the dates and events of the Civil War, or comprehend historical material. For work, we need to learn how to analyze a complex annual report. It takes consistent experience with these tasks and positive feedback, both internal and external, to help us secure these procedures. With success, we come to believe that there is a payoff to engaging the executive and using strategies.

Motivation, self-esteem, and the ability to sustain effort and attention are all variables that contribute to the development and use of meta skills. Individuals who have learning disabilities have been described as having low self-esteem, and/or "learned helplessness." Some of the research in this area indicates that the symptoms of passivity and dependency are the result of negative experiences, such as repeated failure and frustration, as well as the belief that success is attributed to factors outside one's control. Consequently, the executive is not called into action. Recently, some researchers have noted that, while individuals who have learning disabilities are indeed active learners, the problem seems to lie in the fact that they are inefficient and not able to monitor and use appropriate strategies. In either case, we see that the executive is not called into action to regulate and monitor performance in various situations and on different tasks.

## A CLINICAL EXAMPLE

Tom tends to listen to the buzz of conversation in the hallway rather than focusing on the professor speaking at the lectern. When learning new facts, he does not generate schemas or consistently select and apply strategies to help him learn and remember information.

Tom also has difficulty with reading comprehension, as does Sara, whose case we have been following. With complex material, like a science textbook or a business proposal, Tom and Sara read the content several times, but may not be aware that they have not constructed meaning or understood what they read. This may be because they did not apply strategies, such as asking themselves questions, paraphrasing, or activating schemas or prior knowledge in order to comprehend and store new information. This also helps explain why they have difficulty retrieving information from long-term memory.

Tom's difficulty processing information greatly compromises his ability to deal with new information efficiently and effectively. In addition, he lacks motivation, suffers from poor self-esteem, and tends to feel helpless and overwhelmed. This negative self-view also interferes with his ability to accurately evaluate his skills and use strategies to help him perform at a more effective and satisfying level.

A variety of instructional programs that incorporate metacognitive theory are now being used by both teachers and tutors to help people like Tom become more insightful and better able to be strategic and work independently. (See chapter 10.)

Success depends primarily on the use of combined intervention approaches and the ability of the individual to take active control by realistically assessing his needs and monitoring his performance. While much of the research on the benefits of intervention has focused on children, we are now fortunately beginning to see studies suggesting positive and lasting effects with adults.

# 5

# *The Right Diagnosis*

*I was evaluated when eight years old, and at that time
the diagnosis was "word blindness." My teachers did
not understand what this was, and even though my
mother read about the disorder in order to help school
personnel, I was treated as someone who was different.*

Sara, who we discussed in earlier chapters, was discouraged by persistent
learning problems that continued to interfere with her work. She had
never been evaluated, and so did not understand why she struggled with
tasks that others found easy. Sara now wanted answers that would help
her at this stage of her life. Should she remain in her current position as a
nurse or finish college? She had completed an associate's degree but now
wanted to continue, which would mean two more years of school.

Sara was ready to seek help, but like many adults who have learning
problems, she was concerned that she might learn that she was not capable of completing a degree or making a change within her profession. But
Sara was also motivated by her daughter's difficulty learning to read in
first grade. She knew that she could help her more effectively if she
understood her own problems.

## SEEKING AN ASSESSMENT

Sara's concerns are shared by many adults who have learning disabilities.
Some of these adults suspect they have a learning disability, some have
had persistent problems but have never been tested, and some need a
more extensive or updated assessment. For all of them, seeking help is a
difficult step to take. How does one go about finding appropriate professionals? One can talk with other adults who have similar problems and
experiences, or contact physicians, psychologists, and special educators

who focus on learning disabilities. Or one can ask for information from advocacy or professional organizations.

Sara was fortunately able to talk with a fellow nurse at the hospital who had her own son evaluated for learning problems in a clinical facility at a nearby college. But even armed with this information, Sara took several weeks to make the call and set up an appointment. Would she find out that she was not "smart"? Would information from the evaluation make it harder for her to deal with her aspirations and goals? In spite of these concerns, Sara set up an appointment, knowing it was the right move.

Sara chose one type of clinical facility, but there are many settings that provide testing for learning disabilities.

## Settings for an Assessment

- School settings. In a public elementary or high school, testing is performed by a team of professionals. The federal law, called the Individuals with Disabilities Act (IDEA), spells out which professionals must be involved in this process, as well as the criteria for identifying a learning disability.
- Clinical settings. Hospitals and some colleges and universities have clinics where people in the community can be assessed for physical, mental health, and learning problems. Testing is performed by a team that represents various professional disciplines, such as psychology, education, speech-language pathology, audiology, psychiatry, and neurology. Psychiatrists and neurologists are generally part of hospital teams. The definition and criteria used by professionals in the mental health fields follow DSM-IV, the classification system used by the American Psychiatric Association.
- Private office settings. Testing is performed by professionals in private practice, such as psychologists or learning disabilities specialists, or by the two working as a team. These professionals follow the DSM-IV or IDEA guidelines.

## Purpose or Goal of an Assessment

The psychologist H. Lee Swanson describes an assessment as a "goal-directed, problem-solving process." With this in mind, the goals of an assessment are fourfold:

1. To develop a current profile of strengths and weaknesses to determine whether an individual has a disability.
2. To provide placement in an appropriate classroom setting for a student, or in a supportive program within a postsecondary school, work site, or community agency for an adult.
3. To recommend supportive and appropriate intervention. This includes instruction geared to the development of skills and strategies needed for school, the workplace, or the activities of daily living, or referral to other professionals. Most professionals agree that intervention is one of the major roles of assessment.
4. To evaluate and monitor progress.

## Types of Assessment

Psychoeducational and neuropsychological assessments have traditionally been used for both children and adults. Both are considered static approaches, meaning that they include standardized tests that measure skills that are in place or have already developed.

Although the neuropsychological approach is gaining in popularity, the psychoeducational approach is used more often. The distinction between the two depends on the training and professional focus of the evaluator(s). Both approaches look at a range of behaviors, abilities, and skills and use the pattern of strengths and weaknesses to diagnose a learning disability or associated problems.

### *The Psychoeducational Assessment*

A psychoeducational assessment is performed by a psychologist or learning disabilities specialist, or the two working as a team. (See appendix B for information on the role and training of the different professionals.)

Both psychoeducational and neuropsychological assessments follow a four-stage process:

**Stage 1:** Pretesting and information gathering.
**Stage 2:** Administration of tests—the heart of the assessment.
**Stage 3:** Post-test stage, analysis of data.
**Stage 4:** Conference: meeting with the individual and, in some cases, with family members.

### STAGE 1: PRETESTING AND INFORMATION GATHERING

In the initial stage, a broad array of information is collected through questionnaires and interviews with the adult being tested, and the family, when appropriate. This information includes the reason for referral, as well as developmental, medical, psychosocial, school history, and work experience. A review of the history provides a context in which to understand the presenting symptoms and problems. For example, a history of academic problems helps to confirm the diagnosis of a learning disability, which we know begins in childhood and persists into the adult years. In some cases, a delay in early language may be associated with an adult's difficulty organizing and expressing ideas verbally. Physical trauma or childhood diseases in the medical history may also contribute to the diagnostic picture.

### STAGE 2: TEST ADMINISTRATION

The assessment includes both standardized and nonstandardized, or informal, tests. Standardized tests are "norm-referenced," which means that test items are administered to a test sample or large groups of children and adults to ascertain the normal range of responses for a particular age or grade level. This standardization procedure allows us to compare an individual's performance on a particular test—say, reading—to the population at large. Standardized tests include specific guidelines, such as directions for administration, scoring, and time allotment. (See the glossary for types of test scores.)

Informal tests are not standardized, and therefore cannot be used for age or grade comparisons. These tests can be either commercially prepared or tailor-made by the teacher or evaluator. They may measure skills that are not included on standardized tests or performance on different types of tests or questions. They also look at an individual's use of strategies and response to diagnostic teaching or instruction. For example, informal tests might use a particular format or open-ended questions based on an editorial from a newspaper to evaluate comprehension, in addition to the multiple-choice format used in many standardized reading tests. To measure strategy use, one might ask the person being tested to prepare an outline before writing, or to demonstrate the use of note-taking skills for reading comprehension.

Psychological testing typically includes a test to measure intelligence or cognitive abilities, such as verbal reasoning, vocabulary knowledge, memory, and perceptual-motor skills. The Wechsler Adult Intelligence Scale-III (WAIS-III) is the most widely used intelligence test for adults.

The psychological battery may also include *projective* testing, which is used to tap personality functioning. The Rorschach Technique and the Thematic Apperception Test (picture cards of people and situations) are two examples of tests used for this purpose. The Rorschach Technique, for example, uses "unstructured" stimuli rather than representations of familiar objects. The test elicits an individual's spontaneous reactions to the ambiguous stimuli. These responses are thought to reflect one's psychological and emotional approach to organizing thoughts, fantasies, or conflicts in narrative form. Test interpretation follows specific guidelines.

The educational part of the assessment includes a broad array of tests to measure skill development in the academic areas, as well as the ability to process and use language. Academic skills include: reading (word recognition, phonological processing, vocabulary knowledge, and comprehension of text), mathematics (conceptual understanding and computational skills), and written expression (organization of content and use of vocabulary and grammatical structure and spelling). Language tests tap auditory comprehension, needed to process classroom lectures or verbal directions, as well as knowledge of vocabulary and the ability to understand and use grammatical structures and rules. Strategy use is for the most part evaluated informally through the use of interview questions and observation of test behavior.

Clinical impressions of an individual's test performance and behavior are an important part of the assessment process, as they contribute to a richer understanding of individual patterns.

### STAGE 3: POST-TEST STAGE

Following testing, the evaluator(s) review all the data from the assessment, which includes background information, test scores, and clinical impressions. Since a learning disability is a heterogeneous disorder, we see different subsets of problems. Thus, the test pattern and clinical profile can look quite different for each individual. Some profiles may be consistent—that is, reading skills are evenly developed—while others represent uneven skills and abilities, or what we call *scatter*.

We can learn a great deal from analyzing the quality of test responses as well as the pattern of scatter. In reviewing the test profile, evaluators ask the following question: Is the variability in performance related to gaps in skill development, test format, question type, or the pressures of a timed test? For example, some individuals do better with multiple-choice questions than with short essays. Others work slowly, and cannot complete the test questions in the prescribed time. The evaluator(s) also look at the quality of test answers. In some cases, we find that verbal or written answers may lack precision or that thoughts and ideas are not developed or do not include enough descriptive information. Some individuals respond impulsively rather than taking the time to process the question and check the answer, or they do not make use of strategies.

A comprehensive report is written by each of the professionals involved in the assessment process. The evaluators synthesize and analyze the information from the assessment in order to develop a profile of strengths and weaknesses. The profile is then used to determine whether an individual has a learning disability. The discrepancy formula is the most commonly used criterion for diagnosing a learning disability. It determines whether there is a significant difference between one's ability, typically measured by an intelligence test, and one's achievement.

Information from the test profile is used to develop recommendations for instruction or other types of intervention. Two types of recommendations are generally provided. The first type focuses on specific guidelines for instruction or accommodations: suggestions for materials, for example, or techniques for teaching skills and strategies. Accommodations might include the use of a tape recorder for meetings or lectures or extended time for tests or work projects. The second type of recommendation provides referral information that might include a support program within a college setting, or a community-based program. When necessary, a referral is made to another professional, such as a psychiatrist or psychologist.

To be effective, recommendations must be a "good fit" with an individual's needs and goals. For example, why did Sara initiate testing? What were the presenting problems, and what information did she want and need in order to benefit from this process? We know that she was eager to pursue educational and work goals. The assessment should help her to understand the nature of her learning disability and to plan realistically to achieve those goals.

Before we go on to Stage 4, let's return to Sara's experience. Sara scheduled an appointment for an assessment, then met with the team members, which in this case included a psychologist and a learning disabilities specialist. They talked with her about her interest in being tested, her work, and her perception of her learning problems. Sara was asked to complete a form that asked about her developmental, medical, school, and work history. The evaluators reviewed the process and the tests that would be used in the assessment, and indicated to Sara that she would be seen by both team members over four to five sessions.

Sara's appointments with the evaluators had been set up four weeks in advance, so that she could schedule time off from work and prepare herself for what she considered to be a big step. The initial meeting had been helpful, as she felt familiar with the setting and comfortable with the professionals with whom she would be working. Nevertheless, as the day approached, she felt less certain, and again questioned her motives and goals. But Sara was punctual for the appointment, and eager to get started.

At her first meeting with the psychologist, Sara shared the fact that she was anxious and afraid she would do poorly. But a good rapport was established, and she was, of course, encouraged to do her best. As the meeting progressed, her anxiety lessened and, although she became fatigued, she felt that the two or more hours of testing went by quickly. She knew that she did not do well on all the subtests of the WAIS-III, the intelligence test, but she was eager to continue.

With the learning disabilities specialist, her tests and tasks were quite different. Some, like reading comprehension and writing, were difficult for her, but she found the mathematics easy, although she had forgotten how to do many of the problems. But she worked slowly, attempting to retrieve the rules for algebraic equations and do her best. She could hardly wait the two weeks until the team conference!

## STAGE 4: CONFERENCE

When the evaluators met with Sara to review the test results and provide recommendations, the psychologist explained that the WAIS-III consists of two scales, the Verbal and the Performance Scale, and yields three scores: Verbal, Performance, and the global Full-Scale score, which is a composite of the Verbal and Performance scores. This Full-Scale score is referred to as one's IQ. The Verbal Scale includes tests such as vocabulary and verbal reasoning, while the Performance Scale includes perceptual and perceptual-motor tasks.

The psychologist described the variability in Sara's performance. For example, while her vocabulary knowledge was strong overall, her responses were inconsistent in quality. That is, some of her definitions were imprecise or unclear. In the performance area, she was particularly good at constructing abstract designs and puzzles, although she tended to work slowly.

The learning disabilities specialist reported that Sara's errors when reading and spelling reflected phonological problems. For example, she spelled *nashun* for *nation*, relying on the phonetic rule, and made sound substitutions, such as *lesiliant* for *resilient*. She also had difficulty blending sounds into words and discriminating between vowels. And she reversed letters. In many cases, it is difficult to identify phonological problems in the adult, as these symptoms often "soften" with age. Yet, Sara's problems were indeed persistent.

Sara's reading comprehension was variable. She read slowly, and testing indicated that her skills were highly dependent on the level of the material and the type of questions used in the test—in other words, she had difficulty retaining facts when the language and meaning became more complex. This was related to the fact that she did not use strategies to help her construct meaning. Her mathematical knowledge was relatively strong, although errors were evident, particularly with fractions and algebraic equations. She found it difficult to begin a writing task, and did not prepare an outline first to organize her ideas. While her writing sample covered the main points, her ideas were not well developed, she repeated vocabulary, and she made many spelling errors.

Sara learned that she was indeed "intelligent" and capable, but she did have a learning disability. The evaluators indicated that her test profile showed a significant discrepancy between her ability as measured by the intelligence test and her achievement in reading and written expression. It was clear that she had many abilities and strengths that would serve her well in her pursuit of a college degree or advancement at work. But she needed help. This help would include instruction in skill development and strategy use, particularly for reading comprehension and writing.

The evaluators explained to Sara that it was likely that her erratic performance at work was related to the fact that she did not use strategies. When fatigued or stressed, she tended to perform her tasks automatically, without evaluating what was needed. Her executive, or hypothetical manager, was not in full control at these times.

The evaluators answered some of Sara's questions about the causes of a learning disability and what impact it might have on her future. They explained that individuals who have learning disabilities display different subsets of problems that range from mild to severe. Sara also learned that a learning disability runs in families, thus clarifying the incidence in her family as well as her daughter's difficulty reading.

Sara questioned whether she would benefit from tutoring at her age. She was also concerned that she would not have time, given her busy schedule both at work and at home. She did not know whether she should complete her college degree. Were her skills strong enough, and would she be able to keep up with assignments, even with help? Did she have the necessary skills to advance in her professional career?

Sara was provided with the names of several learning disabilities specialists, who were experienced working with adults and who made themselves available in the evening or on weekends. She was also given the names of several colleges that offered support programs for students with learning disabilities. Sara was concerned about sharing the information with other professionals, but was assured that the assessment information was needed both for admission into a college support program and for her work with a specialist. She was also assured of her rights under the Family Education/Rights/Privacy Act (1974), which gives her control over the material.

Sara left the conference feeling both elated and scared. While she understood more about the disability and was assured that she could continue her education and further her professional goals, the thought of getting help, and going on to college, was daunting. She knew that it would have been safer to remain in a job that she knew well. But her assessment convinced her that she should take an active role in trying to achieve her goals.

### *The Neuropsychological Assessment*

There has been an increase in the use of neuropsychological testing over the past ten to fifteen years. This trend has been related to the following factors: (1) advances in research in the neurosciences, (2) the development of new instruments that can localize specific areas of the brain that control functions such as learning and memory, and (3) the classification of learning disabilities as a central nervous system disorder.

The neuropsychological assessment is used to diagnose developmental problems, like learning disabilities, as well as acquired problems, like stroke or head injury. It is also used as a means of collecting descriptive information and clinical data to support research in these areas.

The neuropsychological assessment includes tests similar to those used in the psychoeducational assessment. For example, the Wechsler Adult Intelligence Scale-III is used, as well as a range of tests that tap sensory, perceptual, memory, and motor functioning. The neuropsychological assessment may include educational testing, but the major focus is not on academic problems seen in individuals who have learning disabilities. Recommendations for academic or vocational planning or tutoring are thus not usually part of this process.

## ISSUES IN ASSESSMENT

### Intelligence Tests

Intelligence tests have been used since the early twentieth century when Alfred Binet, a French scientist, was commissioned by the Minister of Public Instruction to develop a way to identify children and place them in appropriate school settings. Binet and his colleagues developed the Binet-Simon Intelligence Scale in 1905 and by 1911 extended the test upward to include adolescents and adults. It was adapted in the United States by Lewis Terman, a psychologist at Stanford University, and became known as the Stanford-Binet Intelligence Scale.

In the mid-1930s David Wechsler, a psychologist working at Bellevue Hospital in New York City, developed an intelligence test that drew on the work of Binet and other psychologists and would become the most widely used test for this purpose. The 1939 version, the Wechsler-Bellevue Intelligence Scale, was developed for adolescents and adults and later named the Wechsler Adult Intelligence Scale. In 1949, the Wechsler Scale was extended downward to include children between five and fifteen years and called the Wechsler Intelligence Scale for Children. In 1967, the Wechsler Preschool and Primary Scale of Intelligence was developed for children ages four through six and a half. These three levels have been revised and updated since that time and are known by their acronyms, WAIS-III, WISC-III, and WPPSI-R.

Intelligence tests are commonly an integral part of the assessment process. They are used in the development of a profile of strengths and weaknesses to determine whether an individual has a learning disability, as well as to predict one's potential to succeed in academic or work settings. While many in the field have questioned its predictive value, studies have shown that intelligence correlates to educational achievement, particularly at the college level. Occupational status and job performance also correlate with intelligence. However, high scores on intelligence tests will not guarantee success in school or work, nor will lower scores negate the possibility of success. While intelligence is one factor, self-determination, perseverance, and metacognition are significant contributors as well.

## Has the Definition of Intelligence Changed over Time?

The work on information processing and metacognition has had a significant impact on the study of intelligence. It is now a generally accepted fact that intelligent behavior is governed to a large degree by metacognition, or our sense of ourselves as learners, and our ability to be strategic. These abilities and skills are not included in the definition or measured in the intelligence tests currently in use, however. While most would agree that intelligence includes a combination of both verbal and nonverbal abilities, many psychologists are now suggesting that we expand the definition of intelligence to include features of self-awareness and problem-solving ability. Some have even suggested that we include executive function, emotion, and creativity.

While intelligence tests have been revised and updated over the years, the format and range of tasks used to measure intelligence have remained relatively unchanged. But before any changes in test format can be made, the definition of intelligence must be reframed and updated. And from the work that is available, it seems likely that intelligence will be defined to include a wider and more diverse set of abilities.

## Alternative Approaches to Assessment

### *Dynamic Assessment Approaches*

Traditional assessment approaches have been criticized for the following reasons: the tests that are included are static, measuring the product of learning, or abilities and skills that have already developed; they do not measure the processes used in learning, or the ability to benefit from instruction; they do not measure executive function or use of strategies.

To address these limitations, dynamic approaches are being suggested as alternatives or supplements to the traditional assessment. *Dynamic* refers to the fact that learning is not fixed at some point in time, but is fluid and responsive to development, the environment, and instruction. Learning, then, is in a process of change.

Dynamic assessment grows out of the work by Reuven Feuerstein, an Israeli psychologist. He believed that cognitive patterns or ways of learning could be modified through the use of "mediation," or training by an experienced teacher. Mediation involves first observing an individual's learning style then providing "insight" as to the most effective strategies for that person and task and then allowing ample opportunities for practice. Feuerstein proposed that this support could be used to modify an individual's cognitive style to the point where rules could be internalized and strategies used flexibly and independently. Feuerstein's theories have been translated into a number of dynamic approaches, all of which emphasize this type of training.

Data from the work on instruction has been positive, as reports indicate that these approaches do enable individuals to integrate and transfer training to tasks outside the experimental setting, and that these gains are maintained over time. Instructional approaches use different types of material, and determine the amount of practice and degree of interaction needed between the evaluator or teacher and student. These variables are subject to the task being taught and the level of support needed. The techniques, some of which are described in chapter 10, have been used with individuals or small groups in varied instructional settings.

At this point, dynamic approaches are not usually part of the assessment process. This is due in part to the fact that we have few tests that adequately tap the use of strategies and problem-solving abilities. And these tend to be informal rather than standardized. We also have not identified and defined the components of metacognition in order to find the best means of evaluating these variables. We do know that testing should be more inclusive and directed toward evaluating individual patterns of strategic use and responsiveness to instruction. While we are beginning to move in this direction, it will take some time before standardized tests and informal measures that measure these skills are developed and integrated into the traditional assessment process.

## PORTFOLIO ASSESSMENT

Portfolio assessment is also considered a dynamic approach. It provides a unique way of evaluating an individual's work, growth over time, and response to feedback and evaluation.

A *portfolio* is a collection of school or work-related materials, compiled over a designated period of time. It can include items like a creative writing piece or an art project (for school), or a marketing proposal or performance evaluation (for work). Collaboration between the student and teacher, or employee and employer, provides the dynamic in which the portfolio is developed. The student, however, has primary responsibility for choosing the items that would have particular meaning and relevance. The student's active role in this process helps to encourage motivation and develops the ability to set and define goals.

Initially, both teacher and student analyze the material and evaluate change. With experience, however, the student develops the ability to critique the material independently and to determine what kind of or how much change is needed. Achieving analytical skills and insight are important features of dynamic approaches.

Dynamic approaches reflect the work in both cognitive and educational psychology that has provided us with a window on how individuals process and store information and use strategic aids in learning. These approaches have particular relevance in work with individuals who have learning disabilities, often described as passive or inefficient learners. If we have better tools to evaluate individual learning styles and responsiveness to different instructional variables, then we are in a better position to develop and provide recommendations that are a good fit. And that is clearly one of the goals of the assessment process.

### *Transition Assessment*

*Transition* refers to the shift from one educational setting to another or to emergent roles in society. It is generally agreed that the significant move from being a student, within a relatively protected educational context, to being an adult, who takes on new and varying roles and responsibilities in the larger community, can be difficult, particularly for those who have disabilities. Success depends on realistic goal setting, with the help of family members and other people who can provide support.

It was not until the 1980s that the transition needs of students with disabilities were formally addressed. The development of transition services was due in part to data showing that high unemployment rates, limited access to higher education, and greater financial dependency were among the transition problems seen in individuals with disabilities. As a result, legislative mandates supporting special education, vocational education, job training, and rehabilitation were developed, providing the impetus and funds for new programs, training, and research. The goal of transition services is to provide assessment and then support for individuals with disabilities within these critical transition years. (Chapters 11 and 12 provide a review of transition planning.)

Transition assessment is a comprehensive process that empowers students and their families by giving them a more active role in working toward well-defined personal goals. The process includes a psychoeducational assessment, coupled with on-site or situational evaluations that take place within a real or simulated educational setting, or workplace or community program. Within these settings, evaluation includes observation of an individual's performance as well as consultation with employers or related professionals. It is believed that a comprehensive approach is the best way to identify individual needs and abilities and provide direction and support geared to academic achievement, vocational success, and personal satisfaction.

More and more adults who have learning disabilities are participating in the assessment process. Some are looking to find out whether they have a learning disability, and others are using the assessment in order to qualify for admission into academic or vocational programs. Still others are interested in finding support services to address specific learning problems or associated psychosocial difficulties.

Adults who have learning disabilities represent a diverse group, as developmental needs and skills change significantly over the lifespan. Some of them have been out of academic settings for years, while others may be completing degrees or thinking of returning to an academic or work setting. The assessment process is a difficult but important first step. While the diagnosis and recommendations for intervention are essential features of this process, the assessment helps the adult become educated about his or her disability. Evidence points to the fact that this knowledge is critical if one is to be proactive and develop a sound and realistic set of personal goals. These goals are different for each individual, and range from working toward an academic degree, seeking advancement at work, participating in a support program, or just looking to develop skills and strategies.

# 6

## *Dyslexia*

*My mother and father always told me I was smart. But
when you work so hard and need to put in so much
more time and effort than everyone else, it's hard to feel
intelligent.*

A friend recently described her experiences when shopping in the super-
market: "I feel overwhelmed by the print, all the letters, all the colors. I
certainly see the print and I can identify all the letters, but I have difficulty
recognizing the words on the boxes. I have to concentrate to locate the
items I am seeking." Sharon, an accomplished woman in her early forties,
was diagnosed years ago as having the learning disorder dyslexia.

School had always been a struggle for her. Outside the classroom,
Sharon had many friends and enjoyed music and art. But at school, she
had a hard time reading and writing. She would write when she had to,
but was always embarrassed by the finished product. It was filled with
spelling errors—including reversals of letters and words, such as *b* for *d*
and *saw* for *was*—and inappropriate word choice. Her handwriting was
poor, too.

> I had lots of good ideas in my head, but I couldn't get them down on paper.
> Spelling was always a challenge. Sometimes I would abandon a particular
> word because I just couldn't figure out the spelling. So I would pick a dif-
> ferent word, one I did know, but, unfortunately, that really didn't fit the
> essence of the paper. Handwriting was an enormous effort. Sometimes,
> when I had to use cursive writing, forming the letters would take so much
> energy and attention that I seemed to have few resources left for thinking
> about the development of ideas.

Sharon's greatest fear was having to read aloud: "In the early grades we
used to sit in a circle and take turns reading aloud. When it was my turn, I

would panic; my insides would churn, my hands get clammy, I would feel myself drenched in a cold sweat as the print seemed to swim before my eyes." Sharon read slowly and haltingly, reversing, confusing, and omitting words, as well as inserting words that were not there.

Fortunately, Sharon was always good with mathematical tasks. Although she did have some trouble mastering basic number facts, her problem-solving skills were outstanding. Her math achievement convinced Sharon that she was not stupid. She had a good academic record in high school, for which she worked very hard, and then spent two years in a trade school. Sharon married, had two children, one of whom has a learning disability, and currently works as a buyer for a major department store.

Sharon still has trouble decoding individual words, particularly made-up words that other people might find easy to sound out. But overall, her word-reading accuracy has improved over time. She still hates to read aloud because it causes her the same difficulty it did when she was a child. On the other hand, when presented with words in the context of a book, particularly a book that taps into her areas of interest, she reads quite proficiently, although slowly. Sharon has learned how to use her intelligence, well-developed vocabulary, general knowledge, and the context of the reading material to help her compensate for her weakness in decoding.

Spelling presents a greater challenge: "I am grateful when my misspellings are close enough to the actual spelling to be picked up by the computer's spellchecker." She makes a few errors that seem phonically reasonable—for example, writing *backaik* for *backache*—but most are nonphonetic, as in the case of *jone* for *join* or *fial* for *final*. Words with several syllables pose the greatest problems. She recalls having written *underlee* for *umbrella*.

While most professionals would agree that Sharon displays characteristics fairly representative of those commonly associated with dyslexia, there is no unanimously accepted definition of this learning disability. Characterized by extreme difficulty learning to read and write, despite conventional instruction, dyslexia was first described by W. Pringle Morgan and shortly thereafter by James Hinshelwood, who named it "congenital word blindness." The term dyslexia—from the Greek *dys*, meaning "disorder," and *lexicos*, meaning "words"—was coined by Rudolf Berlin in 1887.

Like all learning disabilities, dyslexia has a neurological base. But there is much we do not know about it. Should every individual who has a learning disability in reading be considered dyslexic? Is dyslexia a unique disorder with different underlying causes than other learning disabilities? Or does reading ability fall along a continuum, so that children with dyslexia differ from one another and from other readers along a continuous distribution?

Most experts do not believe that every individual experiencing difficulty with reading is dyslexic, but it is often difficult in a classroom or remedial setting to distinguish between the symptoms of the person who is dyslexic and the "garden-variety poor reader"—a phrase used in the literature to describe individuals who have difficulty learning to read for a variety of reasons, possibly as part of a more extensive set of problems that involves mathematics, listening, and perhaps a borderline IQ. For these individuals, reading achievement and intellectual potential may be fairly comparable. In practice, an individual with dyslexia does not always display a discrete set of characteristics easily distinguishable from those of other poor readers. Even phonological issues may not be unique to the dyslexic. We may need to look for other factors or, perhaps, a specific constellation of traits that still needs to be identified.

Dyslexia, like other learning disabilities, is defined by criteria specified in federal law and DSM-IV. In schools, youngsters who exhibit the symptoms of dyslexia would be labeled learning disabled according to the guidelines in the federal law. In clinics or hospitals, it is likely that such individuals would be diagnosed as having a reading disorder and, perhaps, a disorder of written expression, according to guidelines set forth in DSM-IV. In both contexts, a diagnosis would be made on the basis of a significant discrepancy between reading achievement and IQ, once environmental factors and sensory impairments have been ruled out.

It is reported that between 2 percent and 8 percent of the population is dyslexic. Because it is hard to define and identify as a distinct learning disorder, an exact statistic is, of course, difficult to determine. Dyslexia tends to run in families. Studies suggest a 45 percent or higher incidence among members of the immediate family—mothers, fathers, brothers, and sisters. While there is strong evidence that genetics plays a role, researchers believe it unlikely that a single gene is responsible. Previously it was believed that dyslexia was more prevalent among males than females, but recent research suggests that the incidence may be fairly comparable across the sexes.

Dyslexia does not correlate with IQ. In fact, highly intelligent people can be dyslexic. Research suggests that dyslexia is caused by a neurological dysfunction that affects cognitive processes essential to learning to read and write. It is persistent; one does not grow out of dyslexia, although remedial support and the development of strategies can help one to compensate for problems.

## THE ROLE OF THE CENTRAL NERVOUS SYSTEM

In order for the complex act of reading to be accomplished successfully, the central nervous system must work efficiently. It follows, then, that some difference in the structure or function of the brain would in some way impede efficient reading. Indeed, there is a great deal of evidence to show that dyslexia results from just such differences. The neurophysiological literature suggests that there is no single feature that distinguishes dyslexia. Rather, it is connected to a combination of possible structural and functional differences.

Early evidence linking a difference in the brain and dyslexia comes from postmortem studies, conducted by Norman Geschwind and Albert Galabruda in the 1980s. Their work with the brain tissues of individuals who had been diagnosed as dyslexic revealed that the two hemispheres of the brain are the same size. In contrast, in the general population, the left hemisphere is somewhat larger than the right. Researchers speculate that this symmetry in the brain results from irregular migration of cells during the sixteenth to twenty-fourth week of fetal development. Although all the brains studied showed this same structural difference, as of this writing only eight brains have been examined.

But modern technologies now allow us to move from postmortem studies to views of the living brain. Computerized tomography and magnetic resonance imaging (MRI), techniques that display visual images of the brain, reveal differences in the left hemisphere of people with dyslexia, supporting the earlier autopsy studies. Brain electrical activity mapping (BEAM), which monitors the brain in action, shows differences in electrical activity produced by the brain primarily in the left hemisphere, as well as differences in the frontal speech zones of both brain hemispheres, in children with dyslexia as they respond to sounds, sights, and words.

## COGNITIVE EXPLANATIONS

Dyslexia is a problem with reading. Reading involves identifying words as well as constructing meaning. Those with dyslexia have a problem, first and foremost, mastering the competencies required for accurate and automatic word identification.

Proficient readers do not skip words as they read. Instead, their eyes fixate on each word at a very high speed. In fact, skilled word identification takes only a fraction of a second. Poor readers, on the other hand, tend to decode slowly and laboriously. This lack of automaticity or ability to decode quickly and efficiently interferes with comprehension. Reading is a highly complex endeavor that requires a high level of attention. And the human brain has just so much attention to allocate during such a demanding task. When word identification is not automatic, a great deal of energy is expended, leaving little energy left over for thinking about the meaning of the text being read.

Historically, the theories defining or describing dyslexia have fallen into one of two categories: one connects it to a visual deficit and the other implicates a verbal or linguistic deficit. Initially, the most common view of dyslexia was that it was due to inadequate visual perception of letters and words. After all, reading begins as a visual task. Over the years research has focused on topics such as eye movements, oculomotor control, visual attention, perceptual span, and processing speed. Today, while scientists generally believe that dyslexic readers' eye movements do differ from those of skilled readers, most see this phenomenon as a *symptom*, rather than a cause, of dyslexia.

Over the past twenty years, the field has largely moved away from a visual explanation of dyslexia, either dismissing it entirely or suggesting that it would apply to only a small fraction of people with dyslexia. Those who discount the visual deficit view cite research showing that dyslexic readers do quite well with visual images alone. They have no difficulty discriminating among faces, pictures, or objects, and can remember letters and words after brief visual exposure to them. Transposing and reversing letters and words are common in the early stages of learning to read and write for dyslexics and nondyslexics alike. And for dyslexics, reversals are but one type of error among many. Dyslexics do have trouble when they try to translate print into speech, as when they have to decode words. Thus, there is a great deal of skepticism surrounding visual deficit theories. On the other hand, there is general agreement and reliable evidence that dyslexia is due to a specific verbal or linguistic deficit, referred to as a deficit with phonological processing.

## What Is Phonological Processing?

*Phonemes* are the basic sound units of a language. These units are used to form words. English, for example, has forty-four phonemes that can be combined to produce hundreds of thousands of words. *Phonological processing* refers to the ability to blend, segment, retrieve, and distinguish among phonemes.

As children begin to read, they must learn to apply strategies to figure out unfamiliar words. Critical strategies are first matching sound to symbol, or "sounding out" words, and then translating a sequence of letters into corresponding sounds, holding these sounds actively in memory, blending the sounds, and ultimately constructing the target word. Each aspect requires phonological processing. Research findings suggest that difficulty with phonological processing underlies dyslexics' problem with word identification.

Processing is what the mind does when it acts like a computer receiving, transforming, retrieving, and expressing information. Phonological processing refers to these operations as they relate to sounds. Discriminating among sounds, taking apart a sequence of sounds, putting them together, holding them in working or short-term memory, retrieving them from long-term memory—all are phonological processing abilities. We can cluster phonological processing abilities into three categories.

The first category, and the one that has received the most attention in the research, is phonological awareness, an awareness that spoken language is made up of sounds and that these sounds have a set sequential order. Phonological awareness involves the ability to break or segment a word into its component syllables and sounds—for example, separating the spoken word *cat* into its three discrete sounds: *c*, *ah*, and *t*. Phonological awareness also includes the ability to recognize and create rhyme, discriminate between sounds, and the ability to blend or put sounds together, for example, merging the sounds *c, ah,* and *t* to produce *cat*.

The second category involves the rate at which we access phonological information; that is, the length of time between looking at, or visualizing, a person, a place, a thing, and saying its name. Individuals with dyslexia tend to have difficulty accessing phonological information stored in long-term memory, so it often takes them longer to produce a desired word on demand. We sometimes refer to this phenomenon as a problem with *word retrieval* or *word finding*, also called *dysnomia*. All of us have trouble with word retrieval now and then—as, for example, when we look at a familiar face and cannot seem to recall the person's name—but this in itself does not signify dyslexia, of course.

Verbal short-term memory is the third phonological processing area. Individuals who have dyslexia do not perform well when presented with tasks that require them to listen, briefly retain, and then repeat verbatim a string of numbers or a series of seemingly unrelated words. This appears to be due to the fact that verbal short-term memory is not working efficiently. Verbal information is held in short-term, or working, memory most effectively when stored in a phonological code—that is, as units of speech rather than as meaningless sounds. Storing information in a phonological code may be difficult to do when phonological processing is impaired.

## Temporal Processing

What is the physiological basis of a person's problems with phonological processing? A current explanation focuses on temporal processing. The word *temporal* refers to timing. A problem with temporal processing means a basic failure of specific areas of the brain to make sense of rapidly changing information. This research suggests that dyslexia is caused by a deficit in specific areas of the brain that interferes with the rapid processing of auditory signals, which, in turn, disrupts the development of the phonological system. The specific areas of the brain involved are not yet identified. We need more evidence before we can draw any conclusions with confidence.

## The Auditory System

This research on temporal processing as it relates to the auditory system has been conducted primarily by Paula Tallal and her colleagues at Rutgers University using language-learning–impaired children. (Dr. Tallal states that more than 85 percent of these children develop reading problems characteristic of dyslexia.) Tallal suggests that children who have language-learning difficulties have trouble processing sounds (both sequences of tones and linguistic sounds) that converge in specific centers of the brain within tens of milliseconds of one another.

Certain linguistic combinations are harder to process than others. For example, sounds from a series of vowels occur in a steady flow lasting for more than 100 milliseconds (a tenth of a second). Phoneme combinations like *m ah* also have a slow transition, perhaps 300 milliseconds between the voicing of the *m* and the *ah*. These sound combinations are not difficult to process. But a vowel coupled with certain consonants, called stop consonants (b, t, g, and p are stop consonants), has a fast transitional period. That is, there is a rapid sound change between the first sound, the consonant, and the second, the vowel. Thus, in a phoneme combination like *b ah*, there are no more than 40 milliseconds between the first sound, *b*, and the onset of the second, the *ah*. Dr. Tallal has stated that for reasons not yet fully understood, the children in her study cannot detect phonemes with rapid transitions. They have difficulty as well with non-speech sounds that have rapid frequency changes.

Tallal reports that these children perform better on discrimination and sequencing tasks when a computer artificially lengthens the interval between one sound, whether a tone or a speech sound, and the initiation of the next. Unfortunately, the human voice cannot extend these intervals. Dr. Tallal teamed with Dr. Michael Merzenich, a neuroscientist at the University of California at San Francisco, and his colleagues to develop a treatment, still in the experimental phase, that uses computer-generated speech to improve the phonological abilities of individuals who have language-learning impairments. Specifically, they designed a series of computer games that artificially stretch out fast transition phonemes. For example, in the phoneme combination *b ah*, the stop consonant *b* would be stretched, resulting in an interval of 300, 400, or even 500 milliseconds instead of just 40 between the voicing of *b* and *ah*. As the children acquire the ability to detect the sound combinations, the interval between the phonemes is gradually reduced.

Whereas to an adult without a disability, the computer-generated speech might sound fuzzy, like someone speaking with his or her mouth covered, children who have language impairments may accurately detect sounds for the first time. At this point, research information suggests that when trained with such a program, the children can recognize differences in sounds that they could not previously detect. They improve in their ability to detect brief and rapid sequences of both speech and nonspeech sounds. Merzenich, Tallal, and their colleagues are suggesting that this treatment may result, for some children, in permanent changes in the brain. We do not yet know whether such training will have an impact on reading ability or help individuals who have dyslexia but are not language impaired as the children in these studies.

### The Visual System

While Dr. Tallal and her colleagues have described the problems children with language learning impairments have processing rapidly changing sounds, other researchers focus on difficulties with processing fast-moving visual stimuli. Some of this work has been done with adults.

Two parallel pathways, called the *parvocellular* and *magnocellular* systems, send information from the retina to the brain. The parvocellular system transmits information more slowly and responds to color, pattern, and fine visual detail. The magnocellular system, when efficient, works faster and is sensitive to global shape, perception of movement, depth, and contrast sensitivity. Researchers believe that the magnocellular system is involved in reading words quickly. It is speculated that in individuals with dyslexia, the parvocellular system operates normally but the magnocellular does not, making it difficult for them to process the visual information that streams in during reading.

The research we are discussing here deals with visual processing, but some researchers suggest that magnocellular neurons may contribute to many other functions of the nervous system, too. Dr. Tallal also suggests that difficulty processing rapid changes in sounds is perhaps part of a more generalized problem processing rapid sensory information—

whether that information is visual, auditory, or tactile. Postmortem examinations of the brains of individuals who had dyslexia do indeed reveal structural differences in the magnocellular system: the cell bodies are smaller and the layers of cells more disorganized than in nondyslexics. So we do know that the parvocellular system in the brains of individuals with dyslexia is similar to that of able readers, but the magnocellular system is not. In spite of this promising research, there is as yet no pervasive and comprehensive data linking problems in the visual system with dyslexia.

## DYSLEXIA IN ADULTHOOD

Sharon's symptoms have varied as she has grown older, but at forty-three her dyslexia persists. Her experience has been typical of individuals with dyslexia. She had difficulty learning to read in first grade, when her formal reading instruction began. Once she managed to acquire basic sound-to-symbol associations, she could "sound out" words of one syllable but not multisyllabic words. Her difficulty decoding words with many syllables has continued into adulthood, and her oral reading is slow and halting. Spelling and other writing problems became evident by fourth and fifth grade. With remedial support, her reading and writing skills improved, although she still has trouble with lower-level skills such as word recognition and spelling. She can read fairly accurately, but slowly and not automatically.

As an adult, Sharon has far more trouble with spelling and writing than with reading. When reading, she relies heavily on context for both word identification and the construction of meaning. And she can read extremely challenging materials when they are of interest to her.

The literature suggests that adults who have dyslexia can succeed and pursue a wide range of occupations. In fact, several studies show that adults who have dyslexia, overall, attain comparable occupational and educational levels to that of the general population. Key external variables—such as type of instruction received in school and degree and quality of remedial support and emotional support, as well as intrinsic factors such as intelligence and degree of disability—affect the success of these individuals. Early identification of difficulties and early intervention are critical in improving reading and writing skills. And if skills are remediated early, it is hoped, secondary problems like emotional issues can be avoided. But even those individuals with dyslexia whose problems are not identified until later in life can be successful if they receive effective remedial support, if they learn and use appropriate strategies, and if they have strong cognitive abilities and motivation.

# 7

# *The Challenge of Reading, Writing, and Mathematics*

*Finding out I was learning-disabled left me with all sorts of questions about myself. Am I flawed? What does it mean that I have this label? Will I have to work extra hard, harder than all the other kids? I did and always will have to work harder to achieve the same results.*

Language development in the early years involves listening and speaking. A child's experience with language coupled with his or her knowledge about the world form the foundation of reading and writing. In cases where language development does not progress normally, it is likely that we will see later problems with reading and writing. On the other hand, it is possible to have what appear to be adequate language skills and yet have trouble learning to read and write.

Research is now suggesting that individuals with reading and writing difficulties, whether or not they have language delays, tend to show evidence of a subtle, specific type of language difficulty, called a problem with phonological processing. Phonological processing, discussed in detail in the previous chapter, refers to the ability to receive, transform, remember, and retrieve the sounds of oral language. Examples would be the ability to segment a spoken word (noting that the word *butterfly* has three parts), or separating a word into its component sounds (fig into *f*, *i*, and *g*), or manipulating sounds within words. Saying the word *cat* without the *c*, or creating rhyme, or noting the difference between words with very similar sound combinations, or blending sounds to construct a word are all phonological processing abilities. However, we would like to underscore the fact that reading and writing are complex acts, and while current research points to a strong link between these abilities and phonological processing, future work may identify other contributing factors.

## MAKING SENSE OF PRINT

Reading is a complex, dynamic process. The successful reader must be a motivated problem solver, actively engaged in constructing meaning. However, meaning does not reside in the text alone. To construct meaning, able readers use background knowledge and experience as a framework for integrating new information.

To perform this complicated activity, the reader must use appropriate strategies to identify the words and comprehend the text and must have adequate levels of attention and concentration. For word identification, for example, the reader might rely on the meaning of the surrounding text to help decipher a puzzling word or phrase. Or, the reader might apply sound to symbol (which we refer to as "phonic decoding") to figure out an unfamiliar word. For comprehension, he or she needs to consider strategies for each of the three phases of the reading process: strategies before actually reading, while reading, and following reading. One might, for example, pose questions prior to reading in order to stimulate one's background knowledge, paraphrase periodically while reading to highlight important points, and summarize afterward, to review and integrate information. Able readers are flexible and vary their strategies, depending on the type and complexity of the material and their own purpose in reading it.

Able readers are fluent readers. They have learned to "break the alphabetic code" and thus can recognize words quickly and easily. On the other hand, if word recognition requires effort and energy, limited resources are left for thinking about the meaning of what one is reading, and understanding is compromised.

For 80 percent of individuals with a learning disability, reading is the major academic problem. Take, for example, Bernard, a thirty-eight-year-old bank manager whose story resembles that of many individuals with a learning disability.

Bernard always wondered why school was so hard. He was told often by his teachers and classmates that it was because he was dumb or lazy, so he came to believe it. He discovered he had a learning disability when he was thirteen years old, after seven years of struggle and frustration with schoolwork.

In kindergarten, he was described as a very verbal, outgoing child, always participating in classroom activities. But his teacher was concerned because he was not mastering the alphabet and he had a great deal of difficulty creating rhyme. (We know that learning the alphabet does correlate with the mastery of beginning reading skills, as does the ability to recognize and create rhyme.)

In first grade, this young boy could not remember and repeat the words his teacher isolated from his reader and presented to him on cards. He would stumble over common words such as *the*, *dog*, and *can*. As the other children recited, "Run Spot, run," Bernard did not know how to respond. Similarly, as the teacher drilled the sounds of the letters, Bernard felt lost. While he seemed to acquire the sounds of the consonants, vowels within words posed a significant challenge. He decoded *cat* as *cut*, *nit* as *not*, and *pan* as *pun*. Mastering the sounds of letters, which we call *phonics*, was harder for Bernard than learning the word as a whole, that is, recognizing the total word by its gestalt. Words recognized by their gestalt are referred to as *sight* words. Children with a learning disability who have problems with reading tend to have even greater difficulty with phonic decoding than with acquiring a sight word vocabulary, although both may pose problems. Both sight word development and phonics are dependent on phonological processing.

Bernard was placed in the lowest reading group and there he remained throughout the first grade. His parents worked with him, teaching him words and the sounds of letters that school year and all summer. His mother was a teacher and thus knew to give Bernard lots of opportunities to practice each skill after it was introduced. His father read to him often, and as Bernard listened and followed along in the books he became accustomed to the flow and rhythm of prose. Because of Bernard's motivation to succeed, his very hard work, the support of his parents, and his intellectual strengths, something extraordinary happened: he entered second grade reading almost on grade level. He had developed a sight word repertoire and had mastered most sound/symbol associations, although his decoding was not yet automatic. His oral reading was still slow and hesitant and marked by substitutions and omissions of words. He dreaded reading aloud. Because of his poor oral reading, he was again placed in the lowest reading group.

Third grade was probably the easiest year for Bernard. He further expanded his sight word repertoire, he learned to break words of several syllables into meaningful units—prefixes, suffixes, and root words (we call this *structural analysis*)—and he learned to use context to help him identify words. In fact, he began to use all these strategies when unknown words interfered with his reading. His oral reading, while improved, remained slow and halting. Youngsters with a learning disability often remain hesitant, somewhat dysfluent oral readers into adulthood. Bernard's third-grade teacher was very supportive and consistently praised his hard work and motivation.

By fourth grade, there was an emphasis on reading comprehension, and Bernard again experienced significant difficulty. In Bernard's day, the major focus of reading instruction in the early grades was on teaching youngsters to decode. It was assumed that if students could decode accurately, comprehension would automatically follow. But in grade 4 students began to read for the purpose of gaining information. Teachers would not usually teach strategies for comprehension but rather would test understanding through a series of questions. Today, in contrast, reading is considered a constructive process in which even the youngest students are taught strategies to assist them in the construction of meaning.

For Bernard, as for all individuals who have problems with reading comprehension, these difficulties might come from more than one source. Bernard had certainly improved his ability to recognize words, and so his decoding was fairly accurate, though slow and labored. Because he spent so much cognitive energy decoding, he had limited resources left to think about the meaning of the text he was reading. Also, because reading was hard for him, he did not read much. This limited exposure deprived him of a broad background of information and the extensive vocabulary needed to construct meaning effectively. Knowledge of the world, as well as knowledge of language such as metaphors, idioms, and complex sentence structure, often comes through experience with reading. Some youngsters have difficulty understanding text, particularly more abstract text, because of limited cognitive ability, or, perhaps, because of overall language problems. Finally, Bernard might have had difficulty with comprehension because he did not apply strategies to make reading more effective.

In middle school, as the complexity and volume of material Bernard had to read increased, so did his difficulties. He struggled to pass subjects that required a great deal of reading and writing. By the eighth grade, his lack of self-esteem had become apparent. Concerned, his parents sought the help of a psychologist, who recommended a complete psychoeducational assessment. Bernard was tested and subsequently diagnosed as having a learning disability. He received counseling to address the self-esteem issues and tutoring to help with schoolwork

With the guidance of the tutor, and a lot of hard work, Bernard learned to use strategies to help construct meaning from what he read. The tutor taught him to vary strategies, depending on the nature and purpose of the task. For example, he learned to construct a diagram of the theme, setting, characters, and plot when he read a piece of literature and create an outline for his textbooks. Nevertheless, Bernard read slowly and often had to reread material several times to identify important ideas.

Despite his difficulties, Bernard was accepted to a small four-year liberal arts college. The strategies Bernard learned in middle and high school became even more critical. Faced with the abstract nature of the reading assignments of his courses and the sheer volume of required reading, he needed to acquire additional strategies and evaluate more critically which strategies would be most effective for each assignment. He also needed to develop strategies for time management. Through trial and error and, of course, much effort, Bernard was able to accomplish this largely on his own but with some help from a few close friends and professors and the college's academic resource center. He would periodically drop into the center, where peer tutors would clarify the content of his more challenging courses and help him revise and edit his papers.

With the support of his family, friends, and professors, and through his own perseverance and innate strengths, Bernard completed college. Because he had to take a somewhat reduced courseload, it took him five years and several summer sessions. Following graduation, he took a job at a bank in a large metropolitan area. After the first year, he received an award as the bank's outstanding employee. Three years later he became a supervisor and today is the bank's manager.

Bernard still struggles with lingering reading problems. He still reads slowly. His oral reading remains hesitant and halting. Luckily, he is rarely called upon to do it. Bernard learned years ago to apply strategies to help him construct meaning from text, so his reading comprehension is fairly good, particularly when the topic is of interest to him. But there are times when he must read long and difficult material for the job. When that happens, Bernard discusses the material with co-workers, learning from their summaries, and uses drawings, diagrams, and flow charts to help him build meaning. Not surprisingly, Bernard rarely reads for pleasure.

"What I regret," he says, "is that I didn't discover my disability earlier. Perhaps my elementary school years would have been somewhat less of a challenge. Perhaps I would have felt smarter. At least I would have understood why I struggled so. To this day, I find it hard to believe that I really am smart." Although he understands his disability, he still faces some difficulties every day.

> It takes me longer to read reports, or any material for that matter. So I have to manage my workload to set aside enough time to read slowly and complete the task. I never read aloud. My math skills are fine; quite good, in fact. And I do use many math skills as an executive in a bank. My interpersonal abilities are strong as well. I work well with my colleagues and have been told that I am a good manager. Overall, being an adult with a learning disability is a lot easier for me than being a child with one. I no longer have to read biology and history texts, write research papers, and take scores of timed tests.

## PUTTING PEN TO PAPER

Writing is considered the most complex form of communication. Like reading, it is an active process. Writers exert effort as they call upon prior knowledge and experiences and the conventions of written language to construct a product that did not previously exist. Like readers, writers also use strategies—before they write, while they write, and after they write—and must have adequate levels of attention and concentration. Also like reading, writing requires a range of competencies such as vocabulary, spelling, handwriting, and the formation of sentences and paragraphs. In order to have the cognitive energy to focus on such higher-level activities as the generation of ideas, organization of content, and the clarity and rhythm of the text, a writer's basic skills must be fairly automatic.

We know that, to at least some degree, aspects of writing, as reading, are compromised if phonological processing abilities are impaired. Phonological processing problems are most evident with spelling as, for example, when the sounds within words are transposed (*tpo* for *top*), or when the sounds within words are deleted (*unblevl* for *unbelievable*). Spelling and word decoding are in some ways similar competencies, although spelling a word is more difficult than reading it. The reason is because, when reading a word, one can rely on multiple cues—the context, the sounds of the letters, the visual configuration—but minimal peripheral cues are available when spelling. So, while individuals who are poor in spelling may be adequate decoders, those who have problems with word identification will certainly have trouble as well with spelling.

Typical of individuals with writing difficulties, Bernard has always produced fairly short writing samples. There are a number of possible explanations for this tendency. Perhaps words do not come easily to him because of a problem with word retrieval. Perhaps he lacks automaticity in basic skills, like spelling, punctuation, or vocabulary, which interferes with the flow of ideas. And maybe it is emotionally painful for him to write. After all, writing is a public act, and individuals who have significant difficulties with it may feel exposed and anxious when they write, fearing that others will ridicule their work.

Compositions of individuals with a writing difficulty often seem more like transcribed speech than literate writing. Their samples appear somewhat unplanned, uninhibited, almost unconcerned with audience reaction. They may contain jargon or slang rather than more formal, sophisticated vocabulary. The ideas may be poorly organized or not fully developed. Whatever their age, their writing resembles that of someone much younger.

Bernard's handwriting is difficult to read. He prints rather than uses cursive writing and mixes upper- and lower-case letters. Bernard types whenever possible. The physical act of writing involves fine motor control integrated with visual perception and, thus, we say it is a type of visual motor functioning. There are other kinds of visual motor activities, like putting pieces of a puzzle together. Since paper and pencil or pen are used when forming letters, we refer to handwriting as a visual motor task within a graphomotor context, or simply, a graphomotor task. While a handwriting problem, sometimes called *dysgraphia*, might accompany other writing difficulties, as it does in Bernard's case, it is not considered the principal issue in a learning disability with writing, since primary issues are language-based.

Bernard has both a reading and writing problem. Do these difficulties always co-exist? We do not know for sure, but we do know that if you have a reading problem you will likely have a writing problem, as the skills needed for reading are also needed for writing. As for the reverse, some claim that a writing problem can exist when reading is intact because writing is a more complex act than reading. Others disagree, and propose that if you look carefully you will always find a reading problem, albeit sometimes undiagnosed, accompanying a writing problem. What happens in many cases, they suggest, is a mild reading problem accompanied by intellectual strength that allows an individual to compensate without remedial support, resulting in reading problems that go undetected. It is much harder to compensate for writing problems.

In Bernard's early school years, his teachers and parents were so focused on teaching him to read that they seemed not to notice that he was having a very hard time with sentence construction, punctuation, capitalization, and, overall, producing cohesive text. In the fourth and fifth grades, when he was required to use more complex sentences structures and to integrate information gained from reading into his writing, his problems could no longer be overlooked.

In fourth grade the curriculum shifted from learning to read to reading for information and then writing about the content. This was an extremely difficult task for Bernard, as it is for many students with learning disabilities, since it taps into both reading and writing problems. To write a summary, of course, one must have appropriately constructed meaning from what one has read, a challenging endeavor in and of itself. Constructing such meaning assumes, among other things, essential background knowledge, vocabulary in the content areas, the ability to understand concepts, particularly abstract concepts, and the ability to relate concepts to one another and to organize them into a classification structure. It requires many higher-order thinking skills, such as hypothesizing, evaluating, analyzing, synthesizing, and problem solving. To write a summary, students must not only face the demands of constructing meaning but must then re-express ideas into written form using technical vocabulary and formal language structures.

Bernard was taught how to write by his teachers and tutors as he moved through the grades. At that time, the predominant method of teaching was what we refer to as a *skills approach*, which begins with a focus on the mechanics of written language. So Bernard was taught to write words, which he practiced over and over again. Then he was instructed to compose sentences and punctuate them correctly. Not until sentence writing seemed to be mastered was Bernard encouraged to compose paragraphs and longer pieces of text. In high school, he was taught a structure for paragraphs and compositions, which he found helpful, and his writing clearly improved over time.

If Bernard were in school today he might still be taught from a skills perspective. But more and more classrooms, as well as remedial settings, are using a *process approach* to writing, an approach that begins with composing text. Writing is viewed as a multiple-step process that moves through the stages of prewriting, drafting, editing, and revising. As they work, children confer with one another and the teacher, reviewing, expanding upon, and critiquing their drafts. Children have ample opportunities to write beginning in the earliest grades.

As mentioned earlier, Bernard went to an academic resource center in college, where peer tutors helped him revise the content of his papers and edit for spelling, punctuation, and grammar. Reprinted here is a composition Bernard wrote for placement into a freshman writing course. He was asked to describe a hero:

Wilt Chamberland has captured the Imagination of millions of young people around the world. He deserves the recognition he gets for many reasons. He is a good role moodle. He promotes healthy behavior in Americas youth, and he is an example of how work and detirmation can lead to success.

Wilt Chamberland has appeared on TV promoting the importance of school. And the importance of athletics leagues or recreational programs for children. He is a very successful basketball player which is what made him start to get a lot of recognition. This is not the reason I think he deserves to get the attention he gets. I think he deserved it because he is aware he can be a role modl to a child and he considers that everything he does will have an effect on them. So he makes most of his desicions in his life accordingly. I only wish that every ones role moddle thought as much as Wilt Chamberland does about the effect they have on children.

Note that Bernard's composition is short and simplistic, given his age, degree of education, and intelligence. He seems to know something about developing paragraphs, constructing sentences, ordering words within sentences, and using punctuation and capitalization, but spelling is a major problem. Words are spelled as they sound, and sometimes spelled differently from line to line. Note, for example, the three different spellings of *model*. Also note the spelling of *determination*, in line 4, apparently reflective of mispronunciation. In the second paragraph, notice the incomplete sentence in line 2, the error with subject-pronoun agreement in line 9, several instances of shifts in verb tense and overall awkwardness in phraseology.

When personal computers came along, Bernard could use a word-processing program to alleviate his problems with handwriting, check his spelling and grammar, and make his finished product look better. But his texts are still short and lack the thematic sophistication of his speech.

At work, Bernard dictates to his secretary, who then types, revises, and edits his letters, memoranda, and reports. Whenever possible, he places memos on voice mail. He is particularly concerned about his persistent problems with spelling, and this preoccupation clearly interferes with the flow of ideas. Whenever he puts pen to paper he recalls his struggles and embarrassments as a child in school and is grateful that he now has a secretary, a computer, and strategies to help him write. Unfortunately, his secretary and his computer are not always available. Bernard recalls an incident when he received an urgent message late one night from a top bank executive to circulate a memo to his employees. His laptop computer was broken, so Bernard scribbled a memo that he intended to have typed and edited the next day. Unfortunately, that rough draft wound up in the hands of several of his colleagues. When they teased him about his bizarre spelling and barely legible handwriting, he was humiliated and flooded with painful childhood memories.

## MATHEMATICS: THE TOO OFTEN
## NEGLECTED ACADEMIC AREA

Bernard was far stronger with mathematics than he was with reading and writing. In fact, other than difficulty mastering the multiplication tables in grade 4 and occasional trouble with math word problems, Bernard's performance in mathematics was well above average throughout his years in school. His academic profile stands in marked contrast to Alicia's. A recent college graduate, Alicia is an excellent reader and writer. She has always had success in all her subjects except those involving mathematics.

Approximately 6 percent of the school-age population has marked problems with mathematics, sometimes referred to as *dyscalculia*. Individuals with learning disabilities who have difficulties with mathematics may have such problems concomitantly with their difficulties in reading and writing or may have problems with mathematics alone, as in Alicia's case. The number of individuals who have problems with only mathematics is relatively small. (Note we are using the term *mathematics*, not *arithmetic*. While *mathematics* refers to all aspects of the study of numbers and their relationships, *arithmetic* applies only to the computational operations taught in schools.)

A number of factors may underlie a learning disability in mathematics: visual perceptual difficulties, including visual spatial problems, oral language problems, and problems with recall. Problems with recall may, for example, underlie difficulty retaining and later retrieving multiplication facts. Visual perception is the mind's ability to recognize and interpret visual information and relate it to past experiences. Visual spatial functioning falls within the scope of visual perception and refers to the perception of visual stimuli as they are positioned in space. A visual perceptual, particularly visual spatial, difficulty affects the acquisition of both lower- and higher-level mathematical skills and may manifest itself in problems with measurement, estimating size and distance, telling time, visually perceiving number symbols and operational signs, and visually perceiving a geometric shape as a complete and integrated entity.

Alicia's problems with mathematics were first noted in second grade. Her failing grades on addition and subtraction quizzes were decidedly at odds with her strong performance in the class's highest reading group.

Her teacher and parents were concerned and referred her to the school's special education committee. After a thorough evaluation the committee confirmed that she had a learning disability in mathematics and recommended support services several times a week.

Alicia was lucky. Although there are many children like her, mathematics has received far less attention from researchers, writers, and clinicians than reading and writing have. Often children's difficulties with mathematics are ignored if their reading and writing skills are strong. Problems with mathematics may range from mild to severe and may involve only mathematical calculations, only language-based mathematical tasks, such as solving word problems, or problems with both calculations and reasoning.

While Alicia's problems with mathematics were not diagnosed until grade 2, there were hints of difficulty far earlier. Her parents recall that as a toddler, she did not enjoy playing with blocks, puzzles, models, or construction-type toys. Although this certainly does not in itself signal a problem with mathematics, we know that children who have math problems tend to avoid such activities. In preschool, Alicia was often stumped by such spatial relationships and concepts as up and down, top and bottom, over and under, high and low. She also had a fragile hold on basic concepts of time. She could not understand or verbalize expressions such as "in a half-hour" and "five minutes from now."

In the first two years of school, Alicia seemed to have no trouble learning to count numbers in sequence or to read and write the numerals that represent the numbers she could count. But other students with a disability in mathematics do indeed have problems with these tasks. They may, for example, not count in the proper order or reverse and transpose digits, for example, writing *5* as ੮, or *32* as *23*. In contrast, Alicia seemed significantly perplexed by tasks that required her to perform one-to-one correspondence—that is, to match one set of objects with another and with the appropriate symbol. For example, when her teacher assigned her the job of distributing books and pencils to her reading group, she always counted out too many or too few. Similarly, some children were left without cupcakes when she gave out treats for her birthday.

Alicia had difficulty making sense of the operations of addition, subtraction, multiplication, and division. In fact, as Alicia's class was beginning long division, she was still struggling with subtraction where exchange (borrowing and carrying) was required. Further interfering with Alicia's ability to add, subtract, multiply, and divide accurately was her trouble recalling basic facts.

Alicia uses her fingers to help her add and subtract. As is the case with other academic areas, when lower-level skills are not automatic—that is, when they require effort and attention—resources for higher-level operations become limited. Alicia also still makes what appear to be careless errors when calculating. She may misread operational signs, adding when subtracting is required, or misalign columns when computing multiple-digit arithmetic problems.

Alicia has never used counting strategies to help her compute. When asked to add 6 and 8, she will use her fingers to count. A strategic mathematician, for whom this fact was not yet automatic, might add 8 and 8 and then eliminate two (use a double) or add 10 and 6 and eliminate 2 (use 10's).

Strategies are needed to solve both computational problems and word problems efficiently. Problem solving is much more complicated than the completion of rote algorithms. It involves a knowledge base in mathematics, the ability to apply this knowledge base to novel situations, and the ability to engage actively in thinking processes. Strategies are essential for effective problem solving. Strategy instruction in mathematics, like in all other content areas, must be personalized to meet individual needs and should include teaching students to set goals, to vary strategies based on the nature of the task, to monitor their own progress, and to modify the strategies they are using if they no longer work. To help her perform word problems, Alicia was taught strategies to visualize the problem, reflect on the question, determine the computational operations involved, estimate the response, and calculate and check. Yet, even with her superior verbal skills and this strategy instruction, Alicia finds word problems confusing.

Solving word problems would be even more of a challenge than it is for Alicia in cases where there are also language difficulties. In order to solve word problems, students must understand number words, such as *one* and *two* or *first* and *second*; understand words that refer to quantitative relations, such as *more* or *less*; understand phrases, such as *take away*, that signal operations; and comprehend the syntax of the word problem. If problems are presented in written form, students must be able to read efficiently, so sufficient energy is available for problem solving.

Students with language and reading difficulties may fail to solve word problems even when they can manage calculations.

It would be expected that Alicia's visual spatial problems would make geometry a struggle, and she indeed failed the subject in high school. Visual spatial issues may also account for her problems with time, measurement, and distance. She could not master the metric system, and still confuses the relationship of cups, pints, and quarts. To this day, Alicia has trouble with directionality. She always gets lost, and cannot estimate size or distance.

With extensive tutoring and hard work, Alicia did manage to pass high school algebra, an abstract subject that is very challenging for many students with learning disabilities. A calculator was of enormous help for this class and for other subjects and tasks that required calculations, freeing her to focus on meaning. She took no further math courses in high school. In college, she attempted an introductory course, but withdrew after two months because of poor grades. She then enrolled in a remedial math course, which she failed. This failure, according to her college's policy, allowed her to petition for a waiver and to be exempted from any more math courses.

Alicia did graduate from college and will begin a graduate program in social work. She does not expect to use much math in her future career but, like all of us, she will need math and math-related abilities in her life. She will need to plan and monitor time. She will need to handle bank transactions and balance a checkbook. She may need to compute percentages for purchases when shopping or interpret recipe measurements when cooking. She may need to compute scores when playing games. Alicia believes that, with the help of her calculator and computer as well as with the strategies she has acquired over time, she can adequately manage the mathematical demands of her life.

# 8

# Attention-Deficit/ Hyperactivity Disorder

*Work meetings are usually a disaster. I am never organized and always seem to say the wrong thing.*

Since the 1970s, there has been an increase in the number of newspaper and magazine articles and popular books on the subject of attention-deficit/hyperactivity disorder (ADHD). Most of the media attention focused initially on the use of medication with school-age children, but of late there has been a shift of attention to the management of ADHD in the adult.

All this attention has brought many questions to the fore, among them: Has there been an increase in the number of children and adults with ADHD and learning disabilities? Is ADHD a new disorder? Most researchers do not believe that the prevalence has increased, and in fact, investigators Jack Fletcher and Bennet Shaywitz suggest that it is neither a fad nor the disease of the hour.

While the prevalence of ADHD in the population may not have risen, there has been an increase in the number of adults seeking diagnostic services and help. This is related to the fact that public awareness and acceptance of ADHD and learning disabilities have made it easier for adults to share their problems and seek help from family members, professionals, or the larger community. And this help is more accessible.

We have also seen significant advances in research over the last few years, which have affected what we know about the causes of both ADHD and learning disabilities. This in turn has led to more refined techniques for diagnosis and treatment. At this point, there is a strong body of evidence indicating that both ADHD and learning disabilities can be treated and managed effectively, with the appropriate combination of professional support. And treatment is effective for both children and adults.

## COMORBIDITY OF ADHD
## AND LEARNING DISABILITIES

ADHD and learning disabilities are two discrete disorders, with distinct symptom clusters. While one does not cause the other, they often are seen together in the same individual. Researchers Barkley, Fletcher, and Shaywitz report that approximately 30 to 50 percent of children with a formally diagnosed learning disability meet the criteria for ADHD. Children with ADHD are also at risk for learning problems, with conservative estimates ranging from 10 to 25 percent, and with more than 50 percent of children with ADHD considered to be underachievers in school. There are no data on adults at this time.

Nonetheless, some symptoms are common to both disorders. These include the lack of a well-functioning executive, difficulty with self-regulation, and inefficient use of strategies. Disorganization, limited attention, and poor self-esteem are also part of the symptom picture. ADHD and learning disabilities must be diagnosed with care, as very different treatment approaches are used for each.

## WHAT IS ADHD?

ADHD is a neurologically based disorder that affects from 3 to 5 percent of the adult population. The cluster of symptoms show up in childhood, when they can range from mild to severe. For many, these symptoms persist in varying degrees into adulthood. Fletcher and Shaywitz point out that ADHD is a variation on normal development. If we think of development as falling along a continuum, then it is suggested that ADHD is part of this developmental line, rather than representing a shift from normality. Other investigators believe instead that ADHD is a distinct medical syndrome, like diabetes or hyperthyroidism.

DSM-IV defines ADHD by the following behavioral symptoms: inattention (distractibility), impulsivity, and hyperactivity. These symptoms must be present or seen in two or more situations or contexts, persist for at least six months, and be severe enough to interfere with day-to-day functioning. Some of these symptoms must be present prior to the age of seven.

There are three symptom clusters or subcategories:

- ADHD combined type, which includes six or more symptoms of inattention, and hyperactivity-impulsivity.

- ADHD predominantly inattentive type, which includes six or more symptoms of inattention and five or more symptoms of hyperactivity-impulsivity.
- ADHD predominantly hyperactive-impulsive type, which includes six or more symptoms of hyperactivity-impulsivity.

There is a common developmental course to ADHD. Symptoms seen in infancy include irregular sleep patterns, increased motor activity, and emotional lability. In the early school years, limited attention and difficulty getting along in a group setting may be evident. In adolescence and adulthood, the symptoms most often described are impulsivity, restlessness, poor self-esteem, and poor social skills.

## PROGNOSIS

While one does not outgrow ADHD, the symptoms are reported to fade in approximately one-third of the cases. Reports indicate that the symptoms of ADHD tend to persist in the more severe cases and those that are comorbid, or associated with other psychiatric conditions, such as anxiety, depression, or antisocial personality disorder.

Dennis Cantwell, a child psychiatrist, after a thorough review of the ADHD research from 1985 to 1995, identified outcomes in three groups of subjects:

- In the first group, 30 percent of the subjects reported that the symptoms faded early in young adult life, leaving no evidence of functionally impairing problems.
- In the second group, 40 percent of the subjects continued to have functionally impairing symptoms. Some reported social and emotional difficulties as well.
- In the third group, 30 percent of the subjects continued to experience ADHD symptoms, along with more serious psychiatric problems such as substance or alcohol abuse or antisocial personality disorder.

## CAUSES

Although the etiology or cause of ADHD is not yet known, researchers have identified biochemical factors and functional areas in the brain that may be involved. There is some consensus that an imbalance in the neurotransmsitters or chemicals in the brain may play a role, since some of them, such as dopamine and norepinephrine, have a significant affect on attention, impulse control, and mood. This line of research, while preliminary, is supported by the fact that specific drugs have been found to affect these neurotransmitters directly and alleviate some of the symptoms of ADHD.

Other studies have focused on electrical activity and blood flow in the brain. Neuroimaging techniques have been used to identify the areas of the brain, such as the prefrontal and frontal lobes, that are reported to control executive function and self-regulation—support for this work also comes from clinical reports that individuals with ADHD do have difficulty using these control functions and strategies. In addition, Bruce Pennington, a psychologist, points out that electrical activity and blood flow to these areas are reduced in children with ADHD.

We also know that ADHD runs in families. Joseph Biederman, a child psychiatrist, and his colleagues at Harvard report that parents of ADHD children are two to eight times more likely to have ADHD themselves. Siblings are at greater risk for the disorder as well. Twin studies have shown higher rates in identical as compared to fraternal twins. Also, more than three to four times as many males as females are affected.

ADHD is not caused by environmental factors, such as child-rearing practices. In some cases, fetal alcohol syndrome, environmental toxins such as lead, and head injury in childhood, as well as pregnancy and delivery complications, have been associated with ADHD. At this point, though, there is little agreement as to their significance. ADHD is not associated with one's level of intelligence, degree of education, socioeconomic status, or ethnic background. However, we do know that these variables can play a pivotal role in the development of both negative and positive patterns of behavior.

## A BRIEF HISTORY OF ADHD

The study of ADHD goes back to the early 1900s. However, its name has changed over time. Children who survived the encephalitis epidemics of the 1920s were left with a postencephalitic syndrome characterized by problems with memory, attention, hyperactivity, and a lack of impulse control. There was also a group of children who, though not postencephalitic, presented clinically with the same triad of symptoms: hyperactivity, impulsivity, and distractibility. The term *minimal brain damage* or *hyperactive child syndrome* was used for this group. However, when it became apparent that there was no frank evidence of brain damage, the designation was changed to minimal brain *dysfunction*, although *hyperactive child syndrome* was also in use.

During the 1970s, it was thought that the focus on hyperactivity was not clinically warranted and did not sufficiently accent problems with attention and impulse control. In view of the latter, the DSM-III revision of 1980 changed the designation to *attention deficit disorder*, with or without hyperactivity, thus highlighting inattention and distractibility. DSM-III-R, the 1987 revision, provided the redesignation *attention-deficit/hyperactivity disorder*, with two types, one with hyperactivity and the other in which inattention was most prominent. In 1994, DSM-IV continued the use of attention-deficit/hyperactivity disorder; however, three subcategories were added. (These are noted in the previous section, "What Is ADHD?")

## SYMPTOMS

### Inattention/Distractibility

Jack was successful in his work as a salesman for a large food company. He was out in the field and able to use his social skills to clinch sales. In school, however, he had a long history of poor grades and problems of which he has painful memories. He was always told to "pay attention," but he could not understand what this meant. He loved to paint and spent many productive hours at this pleasurable work, but when faced with reading or other academic activities, he could not stay focused. He always intended to complete his assignments, but without control and organizational skills he was never able to begin a research project or sustain attention long enough to pull the facts together coherently.

The symptom of inattention, or distractibility, includes difficulty controlling or maintaining attention, task focus, and concentration. One's level of inattention can vary considerably as both internal needs and the demands of a job or task change. Jack was able at times to block out interfering stimuli, but at other times he was bothered or distracted by the intrusion of thoughts or fantasies, or by the noises around him.

Many individuals report that they, like Jack, are able to get things started, but cannot complete a novel, a long work project or report, or even a newspaper article, particularly when the material is uninteresting or difficult. Inattention can also become a problem during lectures or long meetings or even in pleasurable social activities, such as seeing a movie or having dinner with friends. Forgetting appointments and special dates or misplacing important papers or a briefcase are also common complaints.

The symptoms of inattention are often evident in childhood, when they can interfere with a range of school and home activities. Teachers may report that a child has difficulty following directions or attending to a story. And as schoolwork increases, the problems become more noticeable. The child has a harder time maintaining focus and organizing and completing complex school assignments within specific time frames. Mismatched buttons, untied shoes, and a messy notebook are also signs of personal disarray that are often seen in children with ADHD.

## Impulsivity

Rick dropped out of college after one semester. He worked at different jobs for short periods of time, but he always had difficulty getting along. He was argumentative and unable to control his thoughts or actions. He was unprepared for meetings, he interrupted his boss, and he made suggestions that were thought to be inappropriate or tangential. When Rick was about to turn thirty, he decided it was time to go back to college. But he encountered similar problems there. Administrators and faculty viewed him as difficult to get along with and "annoying."

The symptom of impulsivity reflects a lack of thoughtful planning and difficulty inhibiting one's thoughts and delaying one's actions. These problems show up in academic and work settings as well as at home with the family. In classes or meetings, individuals with impulsivity often interrupt or redirect questions, or respond quickly, with insufficient processing or thought given to the content or purpose of the setting. Impulsivity and poorly thought-out decisions can jeopardize everything from personal relationships to a job interview. Individuals who are impulsive are often thought to be self-centered or lacking interest or concern for others.

Impulsive children are often described as impatient or as having a low frustration tolerance. They have difficulty waiting their turn or delaying their own gratification. They interrupt a lot in the classroom and often make inappropriate comments. Recent reports indicate a higher rate of personal injuries among children and adolescents with ADHD, as they act impulsively, without thinking of their own or others' personal safety.

## Hyperactivity

Rick was also hyperactive. In college, he found it difficult to sit through a class or an examination. Even when working with a tutor in the college's support program, he needed breaks and the freedom to move about. He found that working out in a gym once or twice a day helped relieve some of this motor tension.

Of the symptoms of ADHD, hyperactivity is the one least likely to persist into adulthood. Those adults who are hyperactive have symptoms that are disruptive and personally troublesome, including motor restlessness, such as difficulty sitting still, fidgeting, and in some cases foot movements, which the psychiatrist Paul Wender considers a stable and consistent marker for hyperactivity. At times, all of us have felt restless in meetings or lectures, or even at dinner with friends, but what is considered hyperactivity as part of the ADHD syndrome is easily distinguished.

In most cases, hyperactivity is noticed at an early age, when it is described as excessive motor or verbal activity. While these symptoms show up in many different settings, they are usually most apparent in the classroom, where the child is expected to pay attention and respond to an imposed structure, such as sitting at a desk or waiting a turn. Some children fidget and exhibit a lack of coordination and poor fine motor skills, while others may show good or even excellent athletic skills.

## Associated Symptoms

Certain symptoms—such as lability (mood shifts), poor self-esteem, and inadequate control of one's temper and anger—are described in individuals who have ADHD, but they are not essential for the diagnosis. In children, we may see more severe behavior and discipline problems. In any case, these symptoms can be quite disabling, particularly as contextual demands build up. (These symptoms are also seen in individuals who have learning disabilities; see chapter 9.)

Mood shifts may appear as psychological responses to the chronic symptoms of ADHD. When present, they make it even harder to sustain motivation, interest, and attention. Individuals can become easily over-whelmed and withdraw in times of stress, for example, if a supervisor is difficult, when tests and papers are due at school, or if children are sick at home and a spouse is away on a business trip.

As a group, both children and adults with ADHD are reported to lack metacognitive insight (see chapter 4), an efficient executive, and the ability to use strategies. Their passivity and inefficient use of strategies interfere with their ability to set and accomplish goals. The attention, organization, and follow-through needed to succeed is lacking. Their poor control affects their schoolwork, jobs, and personal and social lives. Just meeting day-to-day challenges is an ongoing struggle for them.

Studies point to the fact that individuals with ADHD are at increased risk for psychiatric disorders, such as conduct, mood, and anxiety disorders. Recent research has also identified a specific subset of individuals with conduct disorders who are more at risk for alcohol and substance abuse. In addition, there is a subgroup of children with ADHD with strong family histories of bipolar disorder who also show symptoms of bipolar disorder. A note of caution is warranted, as work on risk factors, comorbidity, and identification of symptom clusters is still inconclusive.

## EVALUATION

No single test can diagnose ADHD. Instead, a trained professional uses the following tools:

- Psychiatric and neurological examinations.
- Structured clinical interviews. These are formulated under different names. One example is Paul Wender's Utah Criteria for diagnosis of ADHD, which includes a review of past history and current functioning.
- Collection of data from informants.
- Additional testing, as indicated.

In the medical or psychiatric examination, which includes the structured clinical interview, both development and current functioning are reviewed: birth history, genetic background, early development, and current medical and psychological status. Since ADHD begins in childhood and is known to run in families, a developmental history can provide evidence about the persistence and duration of the person's symptoms. A positive family history will strengthen the conviction about the diagnosis. It is essential to diagnose any other medical conditions, particularly if drug treatment is indicated or recommended.

A neurological examination should be part of the process in order to rule out neurological disorders.

A careful review of the patient's profile is needed, particularly since ADHD is a heterogeneous disorder, meaning that it includes different symptom clusters. ADHD is also comorbid with learning disabilities and other psychiatric problems. A physician must diagnose ADHD and differentiate it from other conditions, such as anxiety or depression. (This is called *differential diagnosis.*)

In some cases, it is difficult to collect background history, since individuals with ADHD are reported to be poor self-observers and therefore poor informants. Rating scales are thus used to collect information from both the primary informant, the patient, and other significant individuals, such as relatives, spouses, friends, or teachers. The data from these scales help to corroborate patterns of behavior that the patient may not even be aware of. Rating scales provide a list of behaviors to be checked off. While most rating scales were developed for use with children, there are now several versions for adults, such as the Utah Criteria for diagnosis of ADHD, which includes two parts: childhood history and adult diagnostic criteria. The adult criteria include symptoms such as concentration, anxiety, mood shifts, and inattention.

A referral for a psychoeducational or neuropsychological assessment may be recommended. Since ADHD and learning disabilities often occur in the same individual, it is important to develop a current profile to see if learning problems are evident. As mentioned earlier, some symptoms— such as an inefficient executive and inadequate use of strategies—overlap, but the disorders are discrete and their symptoms must be clearly differentiated, so that treatment and intervention are appropriate.

## TREATMENT

While there is no cure for ADHD, several recommended treatment approaches are being used and reported to be highly effective in reducing and managing symptoms. Treatment is considered to be most effective when a combination of therapies are provided and coordinated. Any treatment must, of course, address the unique needs of each individual.

The recommended steps and approaches include:

- Consultation and evaluation
- Education about ADHD
- Medication
- Psychotherapy or counseling
- Support groups
- Social skills training
- Behavioral management
- Vocational counseling

Consultation with a trained professional is the first step in the process. This may be a difficult step to take, but information about ADHD is needed before one can consider getting help. Talking with a professional is useful in many ways. During this time, one can share concerns and ask questions. The professional can provide information about the disorder as well as referral options for appropriate care if the symptoms are suggestive of ADHD.

A comprehensive evaluation is used to diagnose the disorder and provide an appropriate treatment plan. But equally important is the responsibility that professionals have in educating individuals about ADHD, and in helping them accept and understand the nature of the disorder. Only when these issues are clearly understood can people who have ADHD pursue help and share information with family, friends, and the larger community.

### Medication

Of the treatment options, medication has been the most reliable and effective and has the longest history of providing benefit. As early as the

1930s, William Bradley, a pediatrician, successfully treated children who exhibited the behavioral symptoms of hyperactivity, or what is now known as ADHD, with stimulant medication. But it was not until the 1970s that stimulant medication became the treatment of choice. Currently, research on the benefit and effect of medication has centered primarily on children, although we are gradually beginning to see an increase in the number of studies with adults. With children, researchers report positive treatment results in approximately 60 percent of the cases. Medication in combination with other therapies, such as focused psychotherapy—that is, therapy that addresses specific issues—promises the best results.

Medication must be targeted appropriately—that is, to carefully diagnosed symptoms—and be well monitored and controlled. With good management of the medication, the core symptoms of ADHD are reduced.

### Types and Use of Medication

Stimulants are the most widely used medication for ADHD, although tricyclic and nontricyclic antidepressants and antihypertensive, antianxiety, and mood-stabilizing drugs are used as well. Methylphenidate (Ritalin), amphetamines (Dexedrine), and Pemoline are the stimulants of choice, although there is some debate about the success rate. Thomas Spencer and his colleagues at Harvard Medical School report that stimulants are effective in reducing the core symptoms of ADHD, such as inattention, impulsivity, and hyperactivity. Paul Wender suggests that stimulants are the most effective medication for adults, while Dennis Cantwell reported that the response rate is more variable in this age group. Nevertheless, when effective, stimulants benefit the core symptoms as well as associated behaviors, such as difficulty maintaining task focus, poor academic performance and social problems. Reports also indicate that with some individuals occupational and marital dysfunction improve as well.

When medication is prescribed, the dosage and timing are individually monitored in order to achieve maximum gains and minimize secondary or side effects. Typical adult doses of Ritalin range from 15 to 90 milligrams per day. As Ritalin is short-acting, it may be taken in intervals of four to eight hours throughout the day. Usually, the patient starts at a low dose, then increases until the maximum therapeutic effect is achieved. Side effects, which can be controlled by proper dosage, include loss of appetite, dry mouth, insomnia (related to when the medication is taken), increase in heart rate, and hypertension. There is also the potential for drug abuse, particularly in those individuals with ADHD who also suffer from other psychiatric disorders.

Drugs such as Imipramine and Desipramine are designated by their chemical structure as tricyclic antidepressants (TCAs). Imipramine was popular in the 1970s, but Desipramine is now the drug of choice within this category. When used, doses range from 25 to 200 milligrams per day in divided doses. TCAs have a longer duration of action than the stimulants, allowing for more flexibility in dosage. Unfortunately, studies with adults are not finding consistent and positive effects of Desipramine on the symptoms of ADHD.

Nontricyclic antidepressants, such as Monoamine Oxidase Inhibitors (MAOIs) like Pargyline, can also be effective. Although research studies with adults are limited, those that are available report moderate gains in controlling the symptoms. Doses vary depending on the drug used.

Other drugs, such as Propranolol (antihypertensive), Lithium (mood-stabilizing), Bupropion (antidepressant), and Clonidine are being used and studied in children, as are the more recently introduced Serotonin Reuptake Inhibitors (SSRIs), such as Prozac. As yet, there have been few studies done with adults.

Research studies are focusing on the use of combined medications, but as yet there is insufficient data on adults. Ongoing research on how and why the different drugs affect the symptoms of ADHD suggests that the drugs increase the flow of specific biochemicals or neurotransmitters in the brain, such as dopamine, norepinephrine, and serotonin. Just how these biochemicals affect target symptoms will require continued investigation.

Is there a downside to taking medication? Is "zombification" the price one must pay for improved performance? The data suggest that there is no downside. Drugs that are appropriately and consistently managed will bring attention, concentration, impulsivity, and disorganization under better control and reduce hyperactive symptoms. Many individuals report that they feel better and experience a heightened sense of well-being.

Research with children indicates that medication improves their ability to focus and maintain attention. Impulsive behavior comes under control, increasing a child's ability to learn and use problem-solving strategies. Positive effects on short term or working memory have also been reported. It is important to note that while the medication does not reverse specific reading and mathematical problems, it does help concentration and attention, permitting more careful and sustained work on these academic tasks. It is worth mentioning again that when children with both ADHD and learning disabilities are treated with medication, therapy, and tutoring—a multimodal approach—the results are most positive. The multimodal approach is the treatment plan of choice for adults as well.

## Other Approaches to Treatments

Psychotherapy or counseling addresses many of the psychological and social issues and problems that often go along with ADHD. Some of these problems are related to low self-esteem, anxiety, depression, or difficulty with interpersonal relationships. Recent work suggests that approaches that focus on solving specific real-life problems are more effective than open-ended, analytical techniques. For example, a therapist, in focusing on a person's difficulty maintaining attention during meetings at work, might ask, What are you thinking about or what seems to set you off at these meetings? The goal of therapy, then, is to make the individual conscious about his or her thoughts and feelings in these settings. With self-awareness comes an increased ability to control one's behavior.

Behavioral management is a technique that helps individuals identify and apply strategies to improve their day-to-day living. For example, one might be encouraged to reflect on his or her strengths and weaknesses in order to pinpoint negative behaviors, such as going to meetings unprepared or disorganized. Strategies, such as using notes or an outline, would be suggested and gradually put into use.

Support groups provide a different type of experience. Adults with ADHD meet others with similar problems and share experiences and management strategies. Vocational counseling is another type of support and is useful in guiding adults toward appropriate job choices and opportunities.

We know that a well-functioning executive, self-regulation, and the use of task appropriate strategies are essential for learning and functioning in all settings. Strategies serve as mediators. They improve organization and efficiency, making tasks easier. They also help people who have ADHD sustain attention and gain the control they need to modify their behavioral symptoms. Here are some examples of strategies:

- Anticipate timelines.
- Initiate a reasonable work schedule.
- Use a daily planner.
- Set up nondistracting environments for work.
- Learn to take breaks and using varied techniques to interrupt the hyperactive symptoms.
- Become more aware of impulsive behavior and situations that trigger such behavior.
- Make a concentrated effort to listen to others at meetings or in social settings.
- Take the time to think and listen before responding.

## LEGAL PROTECTION

ADHD is considered a handicapping condition, so individuals of any age who have it are afforded protection under the guidelines of Section 504 of the Rehabilitation Act of 1973, and the Americans with Disabilities Act of 1990. (These laws are discussed more fully in appendix A.) Both laws require that postsecondary institutions and employers make "reasonable" accommodations for individuals with disabilities. In academic settings, these accommodations might include untimed testing, taped textbooks, or allowing a student to tape a lecture or to take an examination a in quiet setting. Workplace accommodations might include extra clerical support, job restructuring, more help and feedback on long-term tasks, or a modified work schedule. When appropriate, one might have the opportunity to use audio and/or video equipment to record meetings. It is up to the individual to request help from the appropriate individual or office. ADHD is not a discrete category in IDEA. School-age children with ADHD can receive special educational services only if they qualify as learning disabled, emotionally disturbed, or otherwise health-impaired.

Ongoing work with both children and adults who have ADHD represents the combined efforts of investigators in the neurosciences, psychology, and psychiatry. Data from this work will provide us with a better understanding of the nature of ADHD and comorbid disorders and the most effective treatment approach for the different subtypes. Some studies are currently looking at:

- Comorbidity, or association of ADHD with other disorders
- Clustering of the disorder in families and genetic origins
- Long-term follow-up on the persistence or remission of the disorder in adults
- The role of the brain and the biochemical system
- The efficacy of drug treatment

# 9

# *Psychosocial Factors*

*I had low self-esteem, could not keep up with friends,*
*and was always a little at odds with the group. . . . I*
*never felt I was as good as others.*

Both Sara and Sharon were successful in their work, were married, and had children. While they were discouraged by their continued struggle with their learning disabilities, they managed to address many of these problems through the use of strategies and by seeking appropriate help when needed.

Daniel, on the other hand, still lived with his parents, even though he had graduated from college and held a part-time job. He had hoped to become a high school teacher, but two applications to graduate school were rejected, and he was afraid to try again. He went to work in his father's business, but left when he did not get along with the staff. He then found a job in a local toy store, where he enjoyed the contact with children. But that job did not last, either. Daniel had to ask for financial help from his family, setting in motion the recurrent pattern of dependency. He was particularly self-conscious with his friends, because he felt ashamed that he was still living at home, while they were out on their own in successful jobs. Daniel lacked confidence and was clearly unhappy, but he did not know how to change his life. He felt overwhelmed and helpless.

Psychosocial problems like Daniel's can be very common in people who have a learning disability, although they are not included in the definition. Such problems can be disruptive not only to one's personal life, but in school or at work as well. The few studies that have been done with adults point to the fact that those who have learning disabilities are at greater risk for psychological and social problems such as heightened anxiety, low self-esteem, inadequate metacognitive skills, and poor social perception or judgment. Moreover, comorbid conditions such as attention-deficit/hyperactivity disorder, depression, anxiety, and conduct disorders are frequently found, with ADHD showing the highest rate of comorbidity.

Some individuals who have learning disabilities are able to achieve and maintain success, while others, like Daniel, have persistent difficulty coping with the disability and its accompanying problems. What accounts for the difference? It has mainly to do with the nature and severity of the disability, the age at which the person was diagnosed, and his or her psychosocial strengths. We also need to factor in the demands that must be faced at school, work, and home and whether the person received any or adequate intervention.

Studies have shown that while the problems associated with a learning disability persist, there are adaptive and positive changes that go along with age. A longitudinal study by Emmy Werner, a psychologist, supports these findings. She followed subjects (learning disabled and controls) from birth through age thirty-two and found that by age thirty-two individuals with disabilities were as successful in their marriages, family life, and work as the control group. Werner suggests that protective factors contributed to this success. These include positive temperamental characteristics, the ability to use compensatory strategies, realistic goal setting, and the help of supportive adults. She also notes that at this critical turning point, these individuals had the advantage of opportunities such as education and employment. Other recent studies have also been helpful in teasing apart the risk and protective factors that enable some individuals who have learning disabilities to be resilient while others are more susceptible to stress and failure.

Susan Vogel and colleagues, one of the research teams studying these variables, list among *risk* factors: the type or nature of the learning disability, the degree to which the symptoms are chronic or severe, comorbidity with attention-deficit/hyperactivity disorder, and other psychiatric problems. Poor social skills, unemployment, and divorce are also thought to make it harder to compensate for and cope with one's learning disability.

Using broad definitions of success, researchers have consistently identified self-determination, control, and the ability to set and pursue realistic goals as critical *protective* factors. Others include: well-developed metacognitive skills, acceptance and understanding of one's learning disability, good communication skills, and the ability to call on family, professional, and community support systems. Studies that define success as related to academic achievement and degree attainment suggest that factors such as socioeconomic status, higher ability level, motivation, and the ability to use support systems are salient.

As Werner reported, some problems soften with age. Others may surface as risk factors change over time. At one stage, a student may have to deal with the stress of schoolwork, while at another must face the responsibility of raising a family or maintaining a business. We all find it more difficult to maintain control and resilience in times of stress, but a learning disability adds to this burden.

Psychologists Barbara Keogh and Thomas Weisner point out that we should not underestimate the critical role that society plays in the development and achievement of each individual's goals. For example, in the United States, education and achievement are currently in high regard. A college degree is considered the ticket to professional advancement. The value placed on education influences all of us as we identify and pursue educational goals or the right careers. Success depends on our ability to weigh these external factors in order to make personally meaningful decisions. The person with a learning disability who is self-directed and able to use support systems will attain success more easily.

## PSYCHOLOGICAL FUNCTIONING

The term *psychological* is used broadly to include cognitive and metacognitive as well as emotional functioning. *Cognition*, or thinking, involves our processing and interpretation of information—whether that information relates to academic or work tasks or to personal experience. *Metacognition* includes our knowledge and insight about ourselves, which affects how we think and learn. This knowledge is used by the executive, the hypothetical mental construct, to develop and plan realistic goals and strategies. Executive control allows us to persevere and monitor our performance until we reach these goals.

Our emotions are naturally occurring responses, both positive and negative, that color the evaluation of our personal experience. Feelings of self-worth, self-esteem, and self-reliance, as well as drive and motivation to succeed, are emotionally toned or colored. These feelings are part of the cognitive and metacognitive systems as well.

The ongoing and persistent problems faced by someone with a learning disability often erode self-esteem, and can lead to frustration and consequently anger and passivity. Lack of self-esteem and persistent failure negatively affect motivation, which we need to initiate and sustain goals. But do the lack of motivation, the passivity, and the poor self-esteem often experienced by those who have learning disabilities *result* from this chronic failure, or are these among the primary symptoms of the disability and therefore one of the *causes* of failure?

Self-esteem is dependent on a strong ego or sense of self. Individuals who have learning disabilities must deal with a variety of negative experiences that can interfere with the development of self-esteem. The expectations and demands of family or teachers can feel overwhelming, or repeated admonitions to "try harder" only make the person feel worse. Individuals who have learning disabilities often *do* work hard, but their work and effort are not effective or fully understood by others. We all need external feedback to verify our own perceptions and provide us with psychological support and reinforcement. For individuals who have learning disabilities, this support is especially critical.

Some may use self-destructive mechanisms to insulate or protect themselves against failure, for example, withdrawing from or avoiding negative situations and experiences. They may refuse to do academic or job-related tasks, delay work on a project, lose assignments, or miss classes or meetings. These defensive behaviors may provide temporary relief by enabling the person to bypass the conflict, or the pain of failure, but the problems remain to be solved. A pattern of avoidance may be set in motion.

For others, hostility and anger may serve as coping mechanisms. The anger and disappointment one feels is externalized. Instead of taking personal responsibility for their failure, they displace or attribute it to a teacher, a parent, or an employer, or an "unfair" test or work project. Take Richard, for example, who had been tutored for over a year and a half, but who found it increasingly difficult to meet deadlines, make tutoring appointments, and keep up with his work. When his academic performance declined, he was angry at himself, but he transferred the blame to his tutor, devaluing her efforts. At other times he projected his anger to his employer, whom he believed singled him out disapprovingly. For some, anger and frustration are internalized, so that self-punishing behaviors, or psychosomatic complaints, show up, such as headaches and stomachaches, that often increase with anxiety.

## Learned Helplessness

Research studies with both children and adults have shown that passivity, or "learned helplessness," is a consistent marker associated with a learning disability. This refers to difficulty taking responsibility for one's academic, work, or personal activities and thus becoming excessively dependent on others for direction, solutions, or strategies. Some studies now suggest that individuals who have learning disabilities are not passive but merely inefficient in their ability to identify and use strategies to make decisions or improve performance.

This passivity and lack of initiative can also be seen as protective mechanisms, as they shield one from external demands and possible failure. Remember that Daniel's "helplessness" allowed him to transfer decision making and responsibility onto his family. Lacking the insight and the strategies needed for change, he was locked into a protective state.

While we consider passivity to be primarily driven by internal factors, we know that it is often tacitly encouraged by family or teachers. They may overextend their help or support, without building on situations that foster independence. In some cases, they may share the fear that their children or students will fail. Daniel's parents were concerned and discouraged by his continued failure, and subsequently, had little confidence in him. While they were well-meaning, they did not help him solve problems or lead him toward areas in which he might have been able to succeed.

Other external factors may also contribute to and reinforce patterns of passivity. For example, individuals who have learning disabilities often take longer to graduate from college, primarily because they take reduced course loads. Or they may be employed in low-paying jobs. Such situations lead to extended dependency on family or friends for financial and personal support. This vicious cycle of dependency may be difficult to interrupt.

## Motivation

Motivation is an essential driving force needed for success. *Intrinsic* motivation involves an internal drive, or need to know more, do better, or participate in a task, "for the sake of it." *Extrinsic* motivation is related to the need to please or perform for others—such as parents, teachers, or employers—and so is less tied to personal goals. It has been said that in the beginning we learn for love, and later we love to learn.

Intrinsic motivation is closely correlated with academic achievement. Nevertheless, we all enjoy external rewards and reinforcement—good grades, a promotion, a raise, praise from others—and the personal satisfaction that comes with success. But why are some individuals who have learning disabilities motivated to succeed, while others appear to lack the drive? Many researchers believe that we develop an internal cognitive map that includes insights, self-perceptions, and interpretations of our personal experience. These interpretations develop from our experience, and we use them to guide and direct our behavior. Attribution and metacognitive theories have been used to explain the relationship between these internal representations and patterns of motivation.

### *Attribution Theory*

According to attribution theory, motivation and self-esteem are directly affected by how we structure and interpret our personal experience, both successes and failures.

Studies on attribution report that there are differences in how individuals respond to school success and failure. Students with learning disabilities reported that they attribute failure in school to low ability, while they attribute success to factors outside their control, such as random luck or an easy test. Their attribution of failure to low ability was internalized and understood as a lack of control over the factors that could make them successful. It may indeed seem pointless to them to try. Repeated failure then can reinforce negative self-perceptions and damage motivation. In contrast, students in this study who did not have learning disabilities attributed success to personal effort, reinforcing positive self-perceptions and goal-setting.

Psychologists Barbara Licht and Janet Kistner review some of the recent studies looking at attribution from a developmental perspective. Reports indicate that in the early school years, children below the age of ten view intellectual ability and success as directly related to how hard you try; with increased effort, the more intelligent you become. There appears to be a shift in thinking, though, from approximately age ten through adulthood. Individuals in this developmental period view intelligence and ability as stable factors that are less amenable to change. In this case, effort is negatively related to ability. It follows, then, that with age, failure becomes a more salient factor.

This developmental perspective does provide us with insight when applied to individuals with learning disabilities. We can easily see how persistent learning problems and failure can lead to negative feelings toward schoolwork in the early years and more lasting and devastating self-perceptions later on. This also helps to explain why these individuals are particularly vulnerable to motivational problems and poor self-esteem. A cycle of failure that often lasts into the adult years is common.

### Metacognitive Theory

Metacognitive theory, as outlined in chapter 4, identifies metacognitive insight, the executive, and strategy use as essential components we need to process information and perform a range of tasks. Metacognitive insight involves the realistic assessment of our knowledge and skills. The executive takes control by assessing this knowledge and the parameters of a task in order to use strategies that are a "good fit," then monitors the plans and strategies until tasks are successfully completed. If not, a new plan is put in place. As we have noted, individuals who have learning disabilities are often described as lacking this metacognitive insight and control. The internal cognitive map we develop includes the organization of both positive and negative experience, along with a realistic assessment of our abilities. Individuals who have learning disabilities have fewer opportunities to experience success and may lack the feedback that is needed to develop this insight.

Many factors contribute to the pattern of success and failure in individuals who have learning disabilities. Attribution and metacognitive theories target some of the psychological and emotional variables that are sensitive to both development and experience. The ability to "reframe" or reinterpret experience along positive dimensions is thought to be critical in helping us negotiate and adapt to a range of internal and external demands.

Nancy J. Spekman and colleagues provide us with a comprehensive description of successful adults who have learning disabilities. These adults are proactive, or able to demonstrate a strong sense of control. Both internal and external factors are present as a support system. Knowledge about and acceptance of one's learning disability, perseverance, and metacognitive insight are significant internal variables. External factors include positive feedback and emotional support from one's family, school, and work community. Mentoring-type relationships with tutors, teachers, friends, employers, or other professionals have been identified as particularly significant. Thus, at each point, individuals need to believe that they can take control, evaluate their needs, and develop appropriate coping strategies. But even with this internal sense of control, external support is needed to verify and reinforce positive self-perceptions. The ability to seek help and accept support have been found to be significant factors in those who succeed.

## SOCIAL SKILLS DEFICIT

David is twenty-three years old. He graduated two years ago from a highly competitive university with a major in mathematics. His grades were up and down, except for mathematics, where his performance has been consistently strong. His IQ score falls within the very superior range. In fourth or fifth grade, David was diagnosed as having a learning disability based on a significant discrepancy between his strong intelligence and his below-grade-level achievement in reading and writing. While his reading and writing problems interfered with optimal functioning in school, of greatest concern was his problem in social settings.

Like Daniel, David lives at his parents' home. Neither he nor his parents like this situation, but David cannot seem to find a paying job. While David attributes his unemployment to the poor job market, in fact the greatest impediment is his difficulty with social skills.

These problems became apparent to his parents when he went away to camp at the age of seven or eight and could not make a single friend. He tried to participate in group conversations, but inevitably would blurt out inappropriate, and sometimes insulting and competitive, comments. His bunkmates would get angry, but he barely seemed to notice. The children ridiculed him and called him names, but he seemed to laugh right along with them, apparently unaware that he was the butt of their jokes.

The same problems occurred at home and at school. When David attempted to interact with his classmates, he was rejected. He was frequently unappreciated by his teachers and rejected by them as well. Through the years, David's mother and father watched him bring home playmates who would seldom return. His parents knew that he did not mean to be hurtful and hostile, but his interpersonal communications were so disagreeable that he was unable to make and maintain friends. Despite their understanding, he had difficulty with his relationship with his parents as well.

People like David, with a social skills deficit, lack social judgment. They seem, to varying degrees, to be unable to understand social situations or to be sensitive to the feelings of others. They cannot judge the moods and attitudes of the people in their environment. They may, for example, share very personal information with a casual acquaintance, or speak to a potential employer in a job interview as if he were a peer at a party. They cannot seem to anticipate the social process, confirm whether people have acted as predicted, and adjust personal behaviors accordingly. This may be because they are unable to pick up social cues, understand how others might feel, read people's faces and body language, and perceive the social atmosphere (for example, whether the mood is hostile or friendly and inviting).

Often individuals with a social skills deficit have problems with an aspect of language that we call *pragmatics*. That is, they do not know how to use language appropriately in a given situation. Pragmatics involves the relationship between the speaker and the listener, which includes behaviors such as taking turns in conversation, staying within a topic, asking pertinent questions, and making and maintaining eye contact.

The literature has described these characteristics in children, but the symptoms last well into adulthood. Indeed, David still has trouble making friends, and he has never had a serious relationship with a woman. His social problems are clearly interfering with his ability to find a job. Research tells us that difficulties finding and keeping a job are among the major complaints of adults with a social skills deficit.

We know that, as a group, individuals with learning disabilities tend to be less accepted by their peers. But do all people with learning disabilities who struggle with social interactions have a social skills deficit? This is a difficult question to answer, in part because there is no generally accepted definition of a social skills deficit, no set constellation of characteristics, and few assessment instruments. In the 1970s, research identified social skills problems as a possible correlate of a learning disability but whether they are a primary feature of the definition is still controversial. Psychologists Kenneth Kavale and Stephen Forness suggest that the most appropriate explanation is that a social skills deficit may co-exist with a learning disability, but is not necessarily caused by problems with learning. The definition of a learning disability, proposed by the National Joint Committee on Learning Disabilities, also refers to social perception and interaction, but then goes on to say that such problems, by themselves, do not constitute a learning disability.

What might cause a social skills deficit? It is suggested that central nervous system dysfunction interferes with the processing of information needed for social perception, social cognition, or pragmatic language skills.

## NONVERBAL LEARNING DISABILITY

Mary, also twenty-three years old, has many of the same social problems as David. She has difficulty adapting to novel social situations and problems with social perception, social judgment, and social interaction skills. Like David, she has difficulty interpreting gestures, facial expressions, and body movements. Mary has difficulty understanding sophisticated humor, and has poor pragmatic skills. Whereas David always interacted with peers, albeit the bulk of his interactions were negative, Mary is a social isolate. With age, Mary has withdrawn more and more from social situations.

Let's look at Mary's profile as compared to David's. Her IQ score is similar. However, on the Wechsler Adult Intelligence Scale-III, David's verbal and performance scores are fairly comparable, whereas Mary's verbal skills are markedly stronger. Her performance abilities, such as visual spatial organization, psychomotor coordination, nonverbal problem solving, and visual perception, on the other hand, are areas of significant weakness.

Academically, Mary's greatest challenge has always been mathematics, both reasoning and calculations, and these problems interfere with certain demands of her daily life. On the other hand, she is good at rote verbal learning, word recognition, phonics, and spelling, to at least some degree attributable to strong phonological abilities. Despite these strengths, reading comprehension is a problem for her.

Mary exhibits the characteristics associated with a *nonverbal learning disability*, a term coined by Helmer Mykelbust in 1975 to describe children who showed significant problems in visual-spatial organization, psychomotor coordination, and nonverbal problem solving. These same children had strengths in rote verbal learning and other areas of language. While the literature has described certain neuropsychological features of a nonverbal learning disability, neither a definition nor diagnostic criteria have yet been developed. Some empirical data suggest that a nonverbal learning disability may stem from disturbances in the right hemisphere that would explain problems in visual-spatial organization, psychomotor coordination, and nonverbal problem solving. Much more research in the field is needed, particularly with adults.

## THERAPEUTIC APPROACHES

### Attribution Training

Attribution training is an intervention specifically geared to modify negative attributions. Licht and Kistner describe this training as helpful in changing individual self-perceptions about success and failure. Training sets up an array of challenges, so that individuals are exposed to different types of problems and solutions. Strategies are developed and applied to these problems or tasks. With practice, strategies are gradually internalized and ultimately transferred to the real world. With success or payoff, self-perceptions change, as individuals gradually recognize that strategies give them the control they need.

There are now many other instructional approaches in use that incorporate attribution and metacognitive theories. These theories are integrated into tutoring, academic support programs, and some therapies. In all cases, the goal is to help individuals become proactive, motivated, and independent. This is accomplished through opportunities for success and help developing a realistic understanding of what one can do and how one can take control.

## Social Skills Training

Individuals who are competent socially master social skills without much thought or effort as they engage in daily activities. Those with social deficits need help learning how to live with and relate to other people. The purpose of social skills training is to help individuals acquire a complex set of behaviors that equip them to negotiate a range of social situations successfully. There are curricula available, some developed for children, others for adolescents, that contain structured sequential lessons that teach social skills through modeling, problem solving, and role-playing activities with lots of practice and feedback.

Candace Bos and Sharon Vaughn suggest that effective social skills training programs must aim to:
1. Teach individuals to solve problems and make decisions quickly.
2. Teach individuals to adapt to new situations.
3. Help individuals develop coping strategies for situations that are emotionally upsetting.
4. Teach individuals to communicate effectively.
5. Help individuals develop the ability to make and maintain friends.

## Other Therapies

Many individuals who have learning disabilities also have other internalizing problems that affect their ability to cope effectively with personal and real-life demands. These include depression, anxiety, and attention-deficit/hyperactivity disorder.

In these cases, the techniques of dynamic (psychoanalytically oriented) or other psychotherapies or counseling are used to help the adult who has learning disabilities understand and deal more effectively with the issues and problems that are of concern. The approach one chooses—whether with a psychiatrist, psychologist, or social worker—should be dictated by the nature of the presenting problem and the goals of the individual. In some cases, family therapy is indicated, particularly since a learning disability affects all family members. Medication may be recommended, but it should be prescribed by an appropriate medical specialist, such as a psychiatrist, in relation to a specific psychiatric diagnosis or targeted at specific symptoms, such as anxiety. Medication will be most effective if it is integrated into the overall treatment plan along with other types of intervention.

# 10

## *Educational Interventions*

*I worry about school all the time. It's always on my mind. No matter how much I study, I never know how I am going to do. I am never quite sure I have learned enough.*

In high school, Marc went to the resource room twice a week to get support with reading and writing assignments. The resource-room teacher helped Marc learn strategies for reading and writing and make use of them in challenging courses like chemistry and advanced placement history. Now in college, Marc is enrolled in a support program specifically designed for students with learning disabilities, where he expects to continue to receive assistance with reading and writing.

Edward, Marc's classmate in high school, is looking for a job in sales. Edward also went to the resource room, much more often than Marc, where he received basic skill instruction in reading, writing, and mathematics. Both Marc and Edward worked on their reading. But, whereas Marc learned strategies like self-questioning, summarizing, and note taking to help him construct meaning from what he read, the focus for Edward was primarily on basic skills remediation. Edward still needs help to decode and spell words. The resource-room teacher taught Edward to sound out words, particularly long words, by breaking them down into syllables and to recognize meaningful units within words, such as prefixes, suffixes, and root words. She also drilled him in common words she hoped Edward would learn to recognize by their appearance. Edward received functional skills instruction (in addition to basic skills remediation) designed to help him get along in the world outside of school: consumer education, banking and money, how to complete application forms. Edward is a highly motivated person. He knows he needs to improve his language arts skills and mathematical competencies to be successful in today's technologically based world of work.

Although Edward has earned a high school diploma and has learned how to acquire knowledge in ways other than reading, he feels insecure about his ability to handle the demands at work that require reading, writing, and mathematics. Edward would like to continue to receive support. By asking former teachers and friends, Edward found a tutor, a special educator trained and experienced in working with individuals who have learning disabilities, to teach him reading, writing, and mathematical skills and strategies.

## READING, WRITING, AND STRATEGY INSTRUCTION

Many individuals who have learning disabilities will continue to need some kind of intervention as they face the challenges of college, the workplace, and daily living. They often need remediation in basic reading, writing, and mathematic skills, as well as instruction in strategies for problem solving, time management, note taking, organization of written material, and textbook reading.

This chapter will discuss educational interventions used to develop reading, writing, and mathematical skills and strategies. Let us briefly distinguish between *skills* and *strategies*. There are both higher- and lower-level skills. Lower-level skills should become automatic and relatively effortless to perform, like adding or subtracting a set of single digit numbers. Strategies, on the other hand, are problem-solving behaviors that generally involve some degree of effort, planning, and monitoring, and are applied to accomplish a learning task. Some strategies are so tied to a task and so well practiced that they take little conscious effort. Others may consist of a series of different strategies used in tandem to perform an intricate learning task. Learning strategies vary greatly in complexity. Knowing that the letter *a* makes the sound "ah" is a phonics skill, but applying phonics skills as well as context clues to figure out an unfamiliar word constitute word-identification strategies. Success in any academic area depends upon the mastery of skills and the application of strategy to support and modify how the skills are used.

Adults can learn skills and strategies in a number of settings. Marc receives strategy instruction in a college support program. Edward works with a private tutor. Instruction is available, as well, in programs within the workplace and within agencies and organizations such as libraries, clinics, government departments, secondary schools, and voluntary literacy organizations.

## Cognitive Instruction, or How to Use Strategies

As we have reported throughout the book, findings from both research and clinical practice indicate that a large percentage of individuals who have learning disabilities lack the metacognitive insight, executive control, and ability to use strategies as aids. While there appears to be a good deal of evidence that passivity or "learned helplessness" contributes to this pattern, recent work suggests that individuals who have learning disabilities are indeed active but inefficient in their use of strategies. Some individuals have limited flexibility to shift plans or use alternative approaches; others have a limited repertoire and tend to use the same strategy for everything, even though it may not be effective.

Inefficient use of strategies occurs most frequently on tasks that require complex processing and high levels of effort and attention. While individuals who have learning disabilities may use strategies to improve their performance, these strategies may not be the "best fit," or they may not be applying the extra effort and sustained attention that is needed. Difficulty with memory tasks is a well-reported symptom of a learning disability. Memory involves the storage and retrieval of all types of information. It is suggested that individuals with memory problems may not structure information in the storage phase, leading to random trial and error searches through long term memory rather than rapid and efficient retrieval. If we use the analogy of a filing system, such individuals have stored the information in a file without headings and without any connection between what they already knew and the new information. The information may be found, but the process in inefficient and time-consuming. This delay certainly interferes in school or work settings, when information must be retrieved on demand.

Research studies have consistently shown that information is retrieved more effectively when it is stored within a schema or network of ideas. *Schemas* are clusters of information on specific topics that include the general or central idea followed by related facts (see chapter 4). To build this network, one must analyze and organize the information to be learned. A network for historical information might include, for example, the schema World War II, followed by headings and subheadings, such as the history of Germany and the social political context of that time. As we add new information, schema are expanded in order to connect new and old ideas. With these maps or organizational formats in place, a memory search can be directed toward the file. Knowledge is useful only if it can be retrieved when needed.

Studies examining the factors that contribute to reading comprehension consistently show that strategies are needed to facilitate comprehension at all levels. We know that comprehension requires active monitoring and the coordination of a range of skills. As the language and ideas in what one is reading become more complex, one must activate schema, maintain high levels of attention, and use varying strategies to construct meaning. These might include using an outline, text notes, or summaries, or rereading the material to gain full understanding.

We know that strategies are needed to improve written expression as well. These include setting up an outline, so that ideas and information are organized, incorporating well-organized notes, and then editing for errors. We need strategies to check mathematical problems, to study for a test, and to prepare for a business meeting. Other strategies help us manage our time, organize notes from a meeting, or set up activities for our family.

But one might well ask, Is the use of strategies a new idea? The use of strategies dates back to the time of the ancient Greeks. Since then, we have learned a great deal about the role of metacognition and executive control and how important strategies are for improving memory as well as learning. With research showing that instruction in the use of strategies is helpful for individuals at all ages, particularly for those who have learning disabilities, there has been a burgeoning of programs that provide this type of training. While these approaches are used primarily in academic and tutoring settings, they are gradually being integrated into the workplace as well.

The early studies on strategy training with children offered little evidence that it could be transferred to other tasks, or that the subjects could maintain and use strategies over time. Recent work, though, shows that instruction can be effective in developing strategies and in helping individuals use them independently.

The broad goal of cognitive instruction is to help develop both declarative knowledge, or what we *know*, and procedural knowledge, or what we *do*. This is accomplished by helping one develop and use insight, control, and strategies to organize new information or retrieve stored facts. Instruction provides intense, long-term practice with varied tasks and well-matched strategies. These tasks may be part of academic courses or real-life situations.

The approaches that have been most effective are those that set up a dynamic between the teacher and student or, in some cases, peer and student. The teacher identifies the strategy and then models how it is used. Such an intervention includes verbal mediation, or self-dialogue, which is considered to be useful in helping to guide one's behavior. A dialogue might include the following script:

*What am I being asked to do?*

*Do I understand?*

*What do I do next?*

Once this sequence is well understood, the student follows the model, using the strategy and the self-dialogue. The student then receives feedback and help with self-evaluation. The teacher's modeling and support are gradually withdrawn as the student becomes able to make decisions and use these mediators independently. As students recognize the advantage of using strategies, they become motivated by the opportunities for success and the insight they gain through this work. (The "reciprocal teaching" technique is a good example of this approach and will be described more fully in the section on reading.)

## Teaching Reading

Some adults, like Edward, may need remediation in basic reading skills to help them recognize and decipher single words, phrases, and sentences. Individuals who have learning disabilities are entitled by law to reasonable accommodations at school or on the job, which might include auxiliary aids that help them circumvent their deficits in basic skills. Listening to textbooks on tape, using grammar and spelling programs on a computer, having note takers or readers, using reading machines, and relying on calculators for mathematical computations are examples of auxiliary aids. So, if individuals can use these aids to bypass reading, writing, and mathematical problems, why invest time and energy in basic skills remediation? While these aids are extremely beneficial and certainly have helped adults in academic and workplace settings, remediation of basic skills allows individuals to become more independent.

Edward's tutor used the information from a psychoeducational assessment as well as data gathered from the first few tutoring sessions to create an instructional plan. Based on the assessment profile, Edward and his tutor collaboratively determined the instructional goals. They decided to enlarge Edward's sight-word repertoire (the words Edward can respond to automatically, based on their overall configuration), secure his ability to analyze words by phonics and structural analysis, and work on speed and fluency. These are all basic reading competencies.

Each skill will be introduced in small segments and at a fairly slow pace. Activities will be structured so that Edward has many opportunities for guided and independent practice. The tutor will provide support and feedback. But the tutor will not work on skills alone. Reading must also focus on the construction of meaning. Listening, reading, writing, and speaking must be integrated within the context of meaningful activities. Edward and the tutor will jointly evaluate the effectiveness of each lesson.

There are a variety of instructional techniques the tutor can use to teach Edward skills. Some tutors introduce new letter sounds and words through a multisensory approach, often referred to as a VAKT method (for visual, auditory, kinesthetic, and tactile modalities). The multisensory approach teaches individuals to read and spell words by repeatedly associating how a word looks and sounds and how the hand and speech mechanisms feel when the word is produced. Individuals hear, say, trace, and write letters or letter combinations in a structured, sequential manner. This approach is commonly used with children with significant reading problems like dyslexia, and some advocate it for adults as well. The ideal approach for the adult might be an eclectic one, with VAKT used in conjunction with other techniques.

The tutor may try out numerous instructional methods before finding one that works effectively and efficiently. It is likely that the tutor will use practical reading materials, such as books, articles, or manuals that Edward needs at home or on the job. The idea is that these real-life materials will enhance motivation. But if Edward seems frustrated because the materials are too difficult, the tutor will select a lower-level text that will allow Edward to be successful but still challenged. (This is referred to as "instructional-level" material.)

It is often recommended that an adult with limited reading skills generate his own written material because it will incorporate language that is important and meaningful to him, and the content will be obviously and immediately relevant. It could be about work, or a piece of news, or any item of interest. The teacher or tutor writes the words as they are spoken by the student, then the text is jointly revised. The revised version is read.

The tutor will encourage Edward to read on his own as much as possible. It is expected that he will select reading material in his areas of interest. Although Edward rarely engages in recreational reading, the tutor and Edward both know that the more reading he does, the better he will be able to consolidate skills and build speed and fluency.

The help that Marc requires will be very different. He does not really need basic skill remediation but does need strategy instruction to help him construct meaning from the textbooks he is required to read. In his support program at college, Marc will meet with a special educator three times a week throughout the semester. He will acquire and practice strategies as he reads and learns the required course material. And the tutor will use interactive techniques as she acts as a model and mediator, guiding Marc through the phases of the reading process.

Marc and the tutor will jointly develop goals. It is the tutor's aim to have Marc become a self-regulated learner—that is, a motivated problem solver actively engaged in goal-directed activities. A self-regulated learner has acquired a repertoire of strategies that he can monitor and use flexibly to achieve his goals. Strategies are developed for the three phases of the reading process: before reading, while reading, and after reading.

The purposes of prereading strategies are to identify the goal of reading; activate, assess, and build background knowledge; and predict content. We know that comprehension is enhanced when incoming information interacts with existing schemas. Thus, it is critical that comprehension instruction build conceptual readiness for new material, alert learners to their existing knowledge base prior to reading, and encourage interaction with print through discussion and questioning. Some students may have the necessary background knowledge. Some may have background knowledge but not realize it. And still others may have a limited knowledge base. It is the teacher or tutor's job to find out what students know, help them build a conceptual background, and teach them strategies for comprehending and storing information. Prereading strategies are also designed to establish the purpose for reading, define ambiguities in the text, and motivate or arouse interest.

Among the most common strategies used to accomplish these goals is surveying. The student looks at the title and subtitles of the chapter, as well as graphs, pictures, key words, and summary statements, and then generates ideas and predicts the content and purpose of the material.

Initially the tutor and student can survey together and the tutor can build background knowledge, if necessary. But the ultimate goal is for the student to apply the strategy independently. The tutor begins by modeling—that is, showing the student how the strategy is performed—then provides feedback and support as the student practices. Gradually the support fades as the student performs independently.

As the learner reads, he or she needs to stop periodically, perhaps after two or three paragraphs, to apply strategies that will help him or her identify the main ideas of text. The tutor may teach Marc to ask himself questions, to paraphrase information, to highlight, to take notes, or to identify key words. Marc may use any of these strategies singly or in combination to help him construct meaning. Each individual learns differently, and the nature and purpose of the task affects learning. So the tutor and Marc jointly determine which strategy or strategies to use for a particular reading assignment.

After he reads, Marc must apply strategies to construct meaning for the whole passage, to reassess the purposes of reading, and to consolidate and apply what he has learned. He may learn to summarize, to outline, to take notes, to map or in other ways diagram information, which he can do while and after he reads. As in the instruction of any strategy or strategy combinations, the tutor begins with modeling, provides many lessons for mastery, and gradually encourages the student to work independently. The student must learn how and when to use strategies and how to monitor success.

Many students and tutors use what we refer to as strategy packages, a coordinated combination of strategies that attend to each phase of the reading process. One such package, used with textbooks, is SQ3R. This method, first introduced in 1946 by Francis Robinson and still very popular, begins with the reader surveying (S), then taking the first subheading and turning it into a question (Q). Subsequently, the reader reads from one subheading to the next, trying to answer his or her own question; "3R" refers to *read* (from one subheading to the next), *recite* or paraphrase the main ideas after each segment, either verbally or in note form, and *review* the entire selection.

Marc's instruction takes place on a college campus, but such help is also available in secondary schools, with private tutors, and through a variety of literacy programs. Because of scheduling issues and the fact that each student is taking different courses, the program at Marc's college provides primarily one-to-one tutoring. But some educators advocate tutoring within a small group. When taught together, students can work as a cooperative learning group, applying strategies and engaging in an ongoing dialogue as they jointly construct meaning from the text. In a group, students not only learn strategies but also feel connected to one another, which can help them develop the motivation and interpersonal skills so critical to success.

Nearly any strategy or strategy package can be taught to students in a small group. One particular strategy package specifically designed to be used within a group is Reciprocal Teaching, developed by Annemarie S. Palincsar and Ann Brown in the mid-1980s. Reciprocal Teaching leads students to acquire and apply four strategies: summarizing, self-questioning, clarifying, and predicting. A unique feature of the program is its instructional method: A teacher or tutor and a group of students take turns leading a dialogue aimed at constructing the meaning of the material they are reading. At the outset, the teacher or tutor models the task and leads the group's activity. As the students demonstrate their ability to apply the strategies, the tutor relinquishes the teacher role and assigns a student to teach a segment of text. The teacher, and the student acting as a teacher, model and provide feedback. Research strongly supports the effectiveness of this program with school-age youngsters. We have also seen the success of this program with adults and are impressed with the degree to which it improves comprehension. (It has been very well received by our students.)

Determining which strategy is most beneficial for any reading task should be a collaborative effort between the tutor and the adult student. The student, with tutor guidance and support, can and should select the strategy or strategies most suitable. To become a self-regulated learner, the student must assume responsibility for his or her own learning. Toward that end, he or she needs to be actively involved in the selection, evaluation, and overall monitoring of strategy use.

There are many individuals whose skills are stronger than Edward's, yet not as well developed as Marc's. They may need some attention to skills and lots of work with strategies. The instructional protocol will vary from person to person. Initial and ongoing assessments will help determine the appropriate instructional plans for each individual.

Neither Edward nor Marc has yet entered the workforce. Research tells us that there are many employees whose literacy levels do not meet their job requirements. The National Literacy Act (1991) defines literacy as "an individual's ability to read, write, and speak English, and compute and solve problems at levels of proficiency necessary to function on the job and in society and achieve one's goals, and develop one's knowledge and potential." Approximately 20 percent of American adults are functionally illiterate. The Learning Disabilities Association of America reported in 1992 that an additional 34 percent are marginally literate. And estimates are on the rise. What was considered an adequate level of literacy in 1950 will likely be considered marginal in the year 2000. It is commonly accepted that the requirements of a particular job determine what constitutes adequate literacy for that job.

While certainly not all workers who have limited literacy are learning disabled, many are. In fact, as many as 50 to 80 percent of adults attending literacy or basic education classes have a learning disability. Employers' concern has given rise to workplace literacy programs in all kinds of businesses and industries. Outside the workplace, literacy programs have also been established in numerous agencies and organizations such as libraries, prisons, government departments, secondary schools, and voluntary literacy organizations.

Any adult literacy program must be uniquely designed for its participants. A workplace literacy program should be integrated into job training and should periodically assess the literacy abilities of the workers. In order to customize a program, job training materials, job manuals, and means and methods of communication within the worksite must be analyzed.

The teaching/learning atmosphere in any literacy program should be risk-free and resemble school as little as possible. A social environment where adults can work cooperatively and help one another is best. Adults need to feel a sense of empowerment and personal ownership of the experience. This can be accomplished, for example, by having them help choose materials and projects, perhaps even create methods and materials themselves. Any program must, of course, take into account the participants' backgrounds, current interests, and goals.

Most workplace literacy programs focus on the specific reading and writing skills needed for job performance, teaching things like technical vocabulary or how to decode, understand, and write job procedures. Programs teach skills and strategies using work-related text, then help the individual to generalize and transfer what he or she has mastered to new materials.

The instructional techniques vary and are often dependent on the background and preferences of the instructor and the participants. Successful instructors are those who are flexible and consider their students as they modify the pace of instruction and select a range of methods and materials. The instructors should receive adequate, specific training in the assessment and teaching of adults who have learning disabilities. Finally, they must be sure their students always know what they are learning, why they are learning it, and how it will be personally useful to them.

## Teaching Writing

Even when reading skills have been remediated, using written language may remain a critical problem for adults who have learning disabilities. Such problems will challenge them in college classrooms, in the workplace, and in managing the tasks of daily living.

Researchers have described specific difficulties apparent in the written work of adults who have learning disabilities: poor organization, poor spelling, inadequate punctuation, repetitive use of syntactic structures, and great difficulty with appropriate word choice and elaboration of ideas. Of course, each individual is unique, and problems exhibited by one person may be absent in another.

Through the years, writing has been taught to both children and adults through a skills approach, a process approach, or a combination of the two. A skills approach views writing as a series of subskills, referred to as the mechanics of language, and presents them in order of increasing difficulty. Teaching begins with these mechanics, such as writing letters, then words, then sentences, then paragraphs and whole pieces of text. Not until one skill is mastered is another introduced. So, for example, students are taught that a well-formed paragraph includes a topic sentence, three to five supporting details, and a concluding sentence. A composition includes an introductory paragraph, a body, and a concluding paragraph.

The process approach to writing, on the other hand, views writing as a multiphase process consisting of prewriting, drafting, revising, and editing. Students begin to compose text at the earliest stages of writing development, always focusing on the message of the written material and always engaged in writing for real purposes. The mechanics of writing are usually taught in mini lessons, and then receive attention during the editing phase. Concern for mechanics is not allowed to interfere with the flow of ideas.

We will describe a writing program for students with learning disabilities within a college setting that has been successful in combining both the skills and the process approaches. Students work on writing on a one-to-one basis with a special education tutor throughout their years in college. The tutor teaches them skills and strategies for writing as they work on actual course assignments. In addition, students enroll in a writing course designed specifically for them.

The goal of this writing course is to create independent, self-regulated learners. Within a supportive environment, frequent and meaningful writing activities are provided. Students are taught strategies for prewriting, drafting, revising, and editing. During the revising and editing phases, students evaluate whether their writing makes sense, covers the topic, and is grammatically accurate.

The major part of the coursework follows a process approach. Students brainstorm, draft, revise, and edit with the help of the instructor and peers. Much attention is paid to the prewriting tasks of brainstorming and organizing. Students are taught to use outlines or semantic maps to help them organize their ideas. We find that the greater the attention paid to prewriting, the easier it is to compose. Much open dialogue takes place in the classroom, and grammatical issues are addressed as they appear in the students' work. Grammar rules are taught and practiced in mini-lessons within the class as well as in the tutoring sessions.

Students' compositions are often based on their reading of short essays, which are discussed in class prior to independent writing to ensure understanding. Students record the important ideas of the essay and come to class with their notes. These notes form the framework for class discussions and are used to organize and provide content for the writing assignment.

Many opportunities are arranged for both peer and self-evaluation. Students read each other's papers, talk about them, question one another, and make suggestions. They meet with a peer editor at least once a week. Each composition that students submit to the instructor is accompanied by a written self-assessment, which follows guidelines they have been given.

This is a prototype of a college writing program for students with learning disabilities. Writing can also be addressed in private tutoring sessions, basic education classes, and literacy programs. As with reading, individuals need to acquire writing skills, like punctuating a sentence, as well as writing strategies, like brainstorming and outlining prior to writing. The curriculum—the particular skills and strategies presented—may be the same across instructional settings. It is not the setting that should guide what is taught but rather the needs of each individual, which should be determined by initial and ongoing assessments.

## MATHEMATICS AND TECHNOLOGY

### Teaching Mathematics

Most of us need some basic arithmetic to meet day-to-day demands. In some cases, one's workplace may require more complex skills and strategies. Mathematics is the essence of an accountant's or cashier's job, but some degree of mathematical knowledge is needed for most occupations. All workers, for example, are likely to want to understand their paychecks, examine how net pay is determined, or check their deductions.

The mathematics instruction students receive in the elementary and secondary grades gets generalized to day-to-day living. How much mathematical instruction students receive typically depends on their abilities and their goals for the future. For those students who have learning disabilities and are planning to go on to college, the mathematics curriculum in high school is likely to be at a higher level than for those not planning to pursue postsecondary education. College-bound students may need to take algebra, geometry, trigonometry, and perhaps precalculus.

For non–college bound students, high school mathematics may be geared largely to practical matters. Students might enroll in Personal Finance, where the focus is on money transactions and management, or Survival Math, covering other kinds of math tasks needed at home and in the community. Some schools offer a series of such courses.

Many educators recommend teaching "life skills" mathematics to all non–college bound students: mathematical problem solving within real-life situations, using basic arithmetical principles and often higher-level math skills as well. For example, students may learn to use concepts of measurement to follow a recipe or to hang wallpaper; or apply the principles of trigonometry to analyze miniature golf or to construct a tent.

A distinct and separate life skills program of study need not be developed. The existing high school mathematics curriculum can simply be augmented to allow a specified amount of time within each class to be dedicated to life skills topics. These topics would be related to the content being covered in class.

If adults who have learning disabilities have not developed adequate mathematical skills and strategies while in school, they can obtain continuing instruction within tutorial settings, basic education programs, literacy programs, or developmental mathematics courses in postsecondary schools. Such programs recognize the importance of mathematics for employment, home and family, leisure pursuits, and community involvement. The instructor should be trained in working with adults who have learning disabilities. The focus of instruction is on reasoning and problem solving applied to real-life situations. Instruction moves from the concrete to the pictorial to the symbolic, and teachers utilize a range of instructional aids such as concrete materials (like blocks, coins, or chips), pictures, and diagrams. Skills must be carefully sequenced so that higher-level competencies are built upon lower-level ones. Mathematical learning requires not only conceptual understanding and application but also the use of strategies for problem solving. As always, assessment of skills and strategies needs to be ongoing.

While we would expect adults who have learning disabilities continuing on to college to have adequately developed mathematical abilities, this is not always the case. Also, those attending college after some time off from their educational pursuits may have forgotten basic rules and operations. Some college students struggle with computations, mathematical reasoning, and application of quantitative concepts. Such students generally register for developmental math courses that review such topics as fractions, percentages, ratios and proportions, and solving word problems. Since a calculator can be used to bypass problems with computations, the emphasis tends to be on reasoning and problem solving.

At the beginning of this chapter, we described Edward, a high school graduate who still needs work with basic skills, including mathematical skills. Edward has a great deal of difficulty with word problems, and when he puts pencil to paper he tends to invert, flip, or misalign numbers. With the help of his tutor, Edward hopes to learn to reason and problem-solve as well as to compute more efficiently. He knows he will need these skills for a job in sales.

## Using Technology

Greg, now an adult, remembers first using a word-processing program when he was in middle school: "I stopped hating to write. When my English teacher told me to revise, I didn't sneer. I just typed away."

Technological instruments help adults who have learning disabilities accomplish a range of tasks for school, work, and leisure. With or without a learning disability, adults with technological skills have advantages in the job market. Clearly, a computer scientist, an engineer, or a programmer needs computer expertise, but some degree of knowledge is also expected for such occupations as a cashier, receptionist, clerical worker, mechanic, or graphic artist. Technological proficiency helps in daily life, too—keeping a household budget, maintaining a mailing list for a community organization, preparing a tax return. In instructional settings, technology should be viewed as one critical component of a comprehensive program, used in conjunction with assessment, remediation, and strategy instruction.

When used to help individuals who have disabilities compensate for their difficulties, technological implements are referred to as *assistive technological devices*. Congress has defined this in public law as "any item, piece of equipment, or product system, whether acquired commercially off the shelf, modified or customized that is used to increase, maintain or improve functional capabilities of individuals who have disabilities." For adults who have learning disabilities, assistive technology can help compensate for problems in reading, writing, organization, listening, and mathematics and thus offer them more independence. Technology cannot cure a learning disability, of course, but it can help bypass certain deficits and thus enhance functioning. The technology selected should depend upon the strengths, weaknesses, interests, and experiences of the individual.

Computers have become very popular as a teaching tool to enhance traditional instruction for all students. Teachers can use drill and practice programs to review and reinforce basic skills, or simulation and problem-solving programs to encourage hypotheses, prediction, and recognition of patterns. Such instruction provides immediate feedback to the student, individualizes instruction for many students simultaneously, gives students undivided attention, allows them to work at their own pace, and creates a nonthreatening and highly motivating environment.

Using a computer with a word-processing program—and such programs vary in complexity and the number of features provided—has helped individuals who have learning disabilities compensate for some of their problems with written language. Spell-checker and grammar-checker features allow the writer to receive assistance with editing. It is so easy to make changes on the computer that one's concern with making errors is alleviated, freeing the writer to work on generating and organizing ideas. And what is ultimately produced is a neat, organized document. Many standard word-processing programs have an outlining feature that can even help, in the prewriting phase, with the sequencing and organizing of ideas: the user brainstorms ideas, and the program creates categories and an appropriate order. A word-processing program may also include a dictionary and a thesaurus.

To use a computer for writing, the individual has to work the keyboard. There are commercially available typing programs that teach keyboarding skills. However, for individuals with motor or visual spatial difficulties, developing keyboarding skills may be extremely difficult, and adaptive technologies may be warranted. For example, key repeat eliminators shut off the repeat function, preventing a series of unwanted characters; key-guards, which are flat boards placed over the keyboard, keep the user from hitting more than one key at a time; large size monitors enlarge the print; and speech synthesizers convert written text into computerized speech.

A speech synthesizer can be an important adaptive device for adults who have learning disabilities for both reading and writing. The written text is presented on the screen accompanied by the artificial speech of the computer, and so the individual can see and hear the text simultaneously. A letter, a word, or a sentence can be presented at a time or a whole screen can appear. A speech synthesizer is a critical component of reading machines.

Optical character recognition (OCR) systems are reading machines. With these, the user can directly input text or any other printed material into a computer through a scanner. Once the text has been scanned into the computer, it is read back by means of a speech synthesizer. Reading machines can stand alone—in which case the scanner, the OCR hardware and software, and the speech synthesizer are built into one device—or all necessary components can be hooked up to a personal computer. The quality and capabilities of reading machines vary greatly in terms of the rate at which text can be scanned, the accuracy of the entries, the range of type styles the system can recognize, the rate at which the text is read back, and the quality of the speech synthesizer.

Another device that can be extremely useful for writing is speech or voice recognition. With this device, the user operates the computer simply by talking to it. Speech goes into the microphone, and the computer writes it.

Tape recorders are not high-tech instruments but, when used to tape lectures, meetings, or books, are useful compensatory aids for those with reading, listening, and/or memory problems. Variable speech control tape recorders allow the user to play back material at faster or slower rates than initially recorded.

We have discussed using technology to alleviate problems with writing, reading, and listening, but software is available as well to help with mathematics and organization. For example, spreadsheet programs provide a way to understand mathematical basics, and scheduling software keeps track of tasks and appointments. A data manager system, to help organize dates and times, can also be purchased as a separate hand-held device.

Adults who have learning disabilities often need direct instruction in using specific technologies. But first it is essential that they understand the purpose of using the device. Is it to teach a specific skill, to supplement subject matter instruction, or as a compensatory strategy to bypass specific deficits? And the adult must recognize and accept the value of its use. The need for the technology should continually be stressed and, if multiple functions are involved, those critical to accomplishing a specific task should be introduced first. Like all instruction for individuals who have learning disabilities, there should be some modeling, lots of opportunity for success, relatively simple and jargon-free language, and continual practice and feedback.

## HOW DO WE ASSESS PROGRESS?

A psychoeducational assessment identifies problems that affect academic performance, skill development, and strategy use and provides recommendation for the type of instruction and support that are needed for individuals who have learning disabilities. These recommendations include the use of specific materials and techniques. While this process sets the instructional plan in motion, an individual's progress and response to instruction must be monitored on an ongoing basis, to be sure that there is a good match and that the individuals needs are being met over time.

As Annemarie S. Palinscar and colleagues point out, the real value in assessment is the ability to *prescribe* the direction and content of instruction. Ongoing evaluation helps shape and modify the techniques and materials to be used. The focus or content of instruction will often shift as academic or work needs change. In some cases, individuals require more help with coursework, or with specific skills they need as a result of a job promotion. For some, the number of instructional sessions may be increased to provide the necessary support.

In setting up an instructional program, both short- and long-term goals are identified. Ongoing evaluation is used to determine whether these goals are achieved. The achievement of short-term goals is reflected in changes on test scores, improvement in specific skill areas, and the ability to integrate and use strategies. The achievement of long-term goals is reflected in an individual's success in coursework over a semester or academic year, admission into a college or graduate program, and ability to change jobs or to feel personal satisfaction in achieving success.

Ongoing evaluation includes both standardized tests and informal, dynamic approaches. Dynamic approaches are considered to be most helpful in evaluating short-term goals, as they are particularly sensitive to individual learning styles. Dynamic approaches are generally interactive, allowing the instructor/tutor to observe how one goes about learning a task, how well new learning is integrated and transferred to new tasks, and what strategies are used before and after instruction. Other informal means of evaluating progress include the use of interview questions and self-reports. These reveal how an individual feels about the instruction or what thoughts or processes are used in planning for a test or preparing for a work project. Rating scales are also helpful in eliciting information from both students and their instructors. Questions on such a scale might ask a student to evaluate his or her progress, or a supervisor might rate changes in a worker's performance over a designated period of time. In some cases, on-site observation and evaluation may be used in the workplace or the classroom to identify the skills and strategies that are needed and the degree to which an individual transfers skills and strategies to these settings.

Instruction and support are most effective when individuals are proactive—that is, when they are able to participate in identifying needs and personally meaningful and realistic goals. Success depends on the quality of the instruction as well as on the individual's ability to sustain motivation, persistence, and effort during the extended time of support.

While we know that ongoing evaluation and monitoring should be part of an instructional plan, there is a lot we still do not know about the variables that contribute to success. For example, how much time should be spent teaching a specific skill? What is the optimal number of sessions or the duration of time needed to achieve instructional goals? And what techniques and materials are the most effective?

The studies that are available with both children and college-age students suggest that instruction geared to the development of both skills and strategies is highly effective. Clinical experience supports these findings. We also see that in addition to improvement in the targeted skills, individuals gain self-esteem and feelings of self-worth.

# 11

## *Learning Disabilities and Higher Education*

*I was not diagnosed with a learning disability until my first semester in college. My political science professor recommended I be evaluated. I had trouble in his class, as well as in my freshman writing class. I felt relieved to finally find out why school had always been so hard.*

Over the past fifteen to twenty years there has been a steady and dramatic increase in the number of students with learning disabilities attending colleges and graduate schools. That number continues to rise. Although incidence figures vary, the U.S. Department of Education (National Center for Educational Statistics) reported in 1986 that approximately 160,000 students in postsecondary institutions, have a learning disability. The Heath Resource Center of the American Council on Education found that the percentage of first-time full-time college freshmen reported to have a learning disability rose from 1.1 percent in 1985 to 3 percent in 1994.

There has been an upsurge of applications to graduate schools as well. Some students who had managed to compensate for their difficulties do not find out they have a learning disability until faced with the rigors of graduate school. Adults who have learning disabilities are the fastest-growing group of college/university students with disabilities.

Why such an increase? Perhaps there are more individuals qualified to attend college than there were in the past because of opportunities provided by federal legislation. For example, the children identified and given services under the implementation of Public Law 94-142, the Education for All Handicapped Children Act, passed in 1975, are now of adult age. Also, there is growing national awareness of the postsecondary school needs of all students who have disabilities, reflected, in part, by the passage of the Americans with Disabilities Act in 1990 and the mandates for transition planning now required for all secondary students receiving special education services.

When we talk about colleges, we refer to both two- and four-year institutions. Among the two-year institutions are the community colleges that have seen an influx of students who have learning disabilities, taking advantage of their open-door policy. (In an open-door policy, all students who have completed high school graduation requirements are admitted, regardless of grade point averages.) A community college is a comprehensive, public two-year institution that offers certificates of completion in vocational and technical fields as well as associates of science or arts degrees. There are reportedly more than 500 community colleges in the United States offering services to students with disabilities, and learning disabilities is the largest single disability category served.

More and more colleges and universities are providing support programs for students who have learning disabilities. We believe such programs are critical. And parents, advocates, professionals, and students are demanding services. Colleges and universities are responding, perhaps, in part, because students with learning disabilities are an excellent source of enrollment and revenue—particularly for institutions that have been experiencing financial crises due to decreases in student applicants and increases in operating costs. Students, parents, and the population at large are recognizing that having a learning disability is a lifelong condition. And so the field of learning disabilities, once engaged almost exclusively with providing services for children and adolescents, is now also concerned with the education and retraining of adults.

Despite the consistent growth in the number of students who have learning disabilities in colleges and universities and the fact that students who have learning disabilities are graduating from high school in record numbers, only a small percentage do indeed pursue higher education. Perhaps this is because the transition from high school to college poses so many challenges. In college, there tends to be greater academic competition, more limited personal support systems, loss of a protective environment, and an assumption of far greater responsibility on the part of the student. Class size is usually larger, and time in the classroom is reduced, as there is a far greater emphasis on independent reading and study time. Studying in high school may mean little more than doing homework, whereas in college it often entails rewriting lecture notes, paraphrasing information from textbooks, and integrating information gathered from a variety of sources.

In high school, homework is often submitted daily, with immediate feedback provided by the teacher. Assignments in college tend to be long-range, as well as extensive, requiring students to schedule their time effectively and monitor their own progress. Often students receive grades no more than two or three times over the course of a semester. Some high school teachers may factor in variables such as effort or level of improvement when grading students with learning disabilities, whereas in college, professors tend to base grades solely on one's mastery of the material.

One of the greatest adjustments faced by students who have learning disabilities is the increased personal freedom college offers. College students make their own decisions about how to allocate time, which classes and majors to select, to what degree to participate in extracurricular activities, and how to balance work and social life. They have a greater amount of free time over the course of a day. No longer is their time structured by parents, teachers, and other adults.

The nature and extent of the support systems change significantly from secondary school to college. The law mandates that secondary school students who have learning disabilities benefit from school professionals who initiate the assessment process, develop an educational plan, and coordinate appropriate professional services. Once students graduate from high school, however, the provisions of IDEA (the Individuals with Disabilities Education Act) no longer apply. Students are now in an environment that demands a much greater level of self-advocacy. It is up to them to seek out services, inform professors of their disability, and decide what services are most appropriate for their needs.

As a group, students who have learning disabilities find it difficult to complete college. In fact, the dropout rate for these students is reported to be 10 percent higher than it is for their peers without learning disabilities. This is not surprising, given the new challenges and the fact that students often find themselves inadequately prepared academically and lacking the proper organizational and study skills and self-monitoring abilities. In addition, social immaturity, poor self-esteem, and a sense of learned helplessness may all have an impact on one's ability to achieve.

There are some indicators that tell us which students who have learning disabilities are likely to succeed in college. Strong grade point averages in college preparatory courses, well-developed reading and mathematical skills, above average intelligence, and extracurricular involvement in high school correlate highly with success in college. Indeed, college admissions counselors, often working with support services coordinators, tend to look at these factors when determining whether to accept a student with a learning disability. They assess grades and whether a student is enrolled in college preparatory and advanced placement courses. They also look at results of recent standardized testing, which typically include reading, mathematics, and IQ scores. Generally, as would be expected, the more competitive and demanding the college, the higher the scores required. Those of us who work with college students who have learning disabilities take these factors into consideration, but we know that equally important are such variables as motivation, awareness, and acceptance of one's learning disability, as well as the ability and willingness to sustain the commitment that college will demand.

Self-determination is a characteristic often linked in the literature to college success. It refers to an individual's ability and willingness to assume responsibility for defining his or her own goals, take the initiative for implementing these goals, and accept the responsibility for accomplishments and setbacks. A college student who is self-determined would be aware of personal strengths and limitations, both academic and social; know and apply compensatory strategies; appropriately express needs to faculty and staff; and independently access essential services and accommodations.

Self-determination is not easy to develop. Lack of self-awareness, a passive and ineffective approach to learning, and low self-esteem—too often by-products of years of struggling with learning problems—create barriers to self-determination. Learning disabilities specialists in high school and college, and sometimes even in the younger grades, are now teaching students self-advocacy skills. Self-advocacy, defined as taking action on one's own behalf, is expected to promote self-determination.

## THE LAW

As previously mentioned, after high school, students who have learning disabilities (as well as all other disabilities) no longer qualify for the mandates set forth in IDEA. Their rights become protected primarily by the regulations in Section 504 of the Rehabilitation Act of 1973. This is a civil rights statute that prohibits discrimination of individuals with disabilities by facilities, including colleges, that receive federal financial assistance. (Virtually all colleges receive some type of federal monies.)

Section 504 defines a handicapped person as one who has a physical or mental impairment that substantially limits one or more major life activities, has a record of such an impairment, or is regarded as having such an impairment. Facilities receiving federal monies must ensure that all their programs and activities are accessible to otherwise qualified handicapped individuals. "Otherwise qualified" has been interpreted to mean that when provided reasonable accommodations, the individual is able to meet academic and/or technical requirements for admission or participation in the program or activity in spite of the handicap. (See appendix A for a more detailed description of Section 504.)

What are "reasonable accommodations?" This is a rather gray area that has spurred quite a bit of debate. Accommodations are considered to be reasonable if they do not fundamentally alter the nature of a program. Examples of reasonable accommodations for students with learning disabilities in college settings might include giving them extra time when taking exams, providing them with readers and/or note takers, administering exams to them in a separate room and/or in a different format, and permitting them to use computers or other technical aids. Determining whether a particular accommodation is reasonable in a given situation should be made on a case-by-case basis. The courts have ruled that there are two circumstances under which a college or university may refuse to grant a particular accommodation. The first is undue financial or administrative hardship. Whether, indeed, a financial burden exists would depend, in part, on the size of the program, the financial resources of the program, and the cost of the accommodation. The second defense is safety. This becomes particularly relevant in medical programs such as nursing, medical school, and optometry. For example, it might be considered "unsafe" if a doctor were unable to accurately decode a medical chart.

While students are entitled to reasonable accommodations, in order to receive such aids or services they must inform the institution of their condition and must make a request to be accomodated. A college will require documentation and may specify that it be recent, that it have been performed by a professional, that it include specific tests, and that it be paid for by the student. The college must consider the civil rights of the individual concomitantly with the academic standards and integrity of the institution.

The Americans with Disabilities Act (1990) extends Section 504 to include facilities not receiving federal financial assistance.

## THE TRANSITION TO COLLEGE

All college bound students go through a planning process as they prepare to leave high school. Typically, prior to even their freshman year in high school, students select a course of study and at least a semester's worth of individual subjects. Throughout high school, they engage in extracurricular activities, hobbies, and sometimes work, all of which help them clarify their own interests and aptitudes. Their guidance counselors help them identify their interests and abilities, set personal, academic, and career goals, and make college choices that match those interests and goals. In the junior year, students and counselors generate lists of college options, and students begin an intensive exploration.

College-bound students who have learning disabilities go through this same process but face additional challenges. They may be college-able but lack the proper academic preparation. For example, they may have cognitive strengths, such as the ability to understand abstract concepts to handle college-level work, but have enrolled in modified courses rather than the more demanding college preparatory subjects. They may not have developed enough independence. They may not have engaged in extracurricular activities, hobbies, work experiences, or career exploration—all basic to goal setting. They may not understand their learning disability, or have low self-esteem, or lack confidence and motivation. They may need help in accepting their disability, as well as in selecting colleges that not only match their interests and abilities but offer adequate support programs. They need *transition planning*.

The idea of transition planning for students who have learning disabilities to facilitate their success in postsecondary settings is not new. The National Joint Committee on Learning Disabilities wrote, in 1984, that many students with learning disabilities can go on to higher education and that, if transition plans are designed and implemented well, those students are likely to be successful.

IDEA formally recognized the need for transition plans and services for adolescents with all types of disabilities in 1990. IDEA, reauthorized in 1997, mandates that beginning at age fourteen and updated annually, all students receiving special education services have a statement of transition service needs regarding courses of study—such as advanced placement courses or vocational education programs—as part of their individualized education program (IEP). Beginning no later than age sixteen, students must also have a statement of needed transition services, including, when appropriate, interagency responsibilities—for example, the involvement of the vocational rehabilitation agency. IDEA defines transition services as a coordinated set of activities, selected on the basis of the student's needs, preference, and interests, that promote movement from school to postschool.

We don't yet have much empirical data to guide the development of transition planning and programming. But we do know that, in order for transition planning to work, students must be actively involved in decision making. An ideal transition planning team would include the student, first and foremost, his or her parents, a psychologist, the guidance counselor, the learning disability specialist, the general education teacher, and perhaps a postsecondary learning disability service provider. The team of student, parents, and secondary school personnel is formed when the student enters high school, and the postsecondary school member is added during senior year.

Transition planning for college-bound learning-disabled students should begin early, no later than age fourteen, to give students ample time to develop the skills and competencies critical for college. Also, if students receive guidance as they move from middle to high school, they might, from the outset, be encouraged to take the most demanding academic program they can handle. Whenever possible, this program needs to be provided in an integrated setting rather in the more restrictive special class. The resource room in middle school, and throughout high school, should be used to teach, among other things, those strategies necessary for effective and efficient learning, allowing the student to handle the challenging coursework. For example, students might learn strategies for constructing meaning from textbooks, for organizing, for drafting and revising papers, and for managing their time.

Transition planning and the subsequent transition services should help clarify for students what it will take to achieve success and independence. Students need to acquire academic skills and learning strategies, know about career options, develop self-advocacy abilities, and overall grow in independence. Transition planning gives students the opportunity to learn more about their personal strengths and weaknesses, to understand the nature of their learning disability, to ask questions, to present ideas, and to identify goals and the actions needed to attain those goals.

During the students' junior and senior years in high school, guidance counselors can help them explore the diverse range of two- and four-year colleges and match interests and abilities to these options. In the junior year, students begin to prepare for the SAT or ACT examinations. Support personnel should encourage them to take these tests with accommodations, such as extended time. The extent to which students take rigorous college preparatory courses will, of course, depend on their postsecondary goals. As Loring Brinckerhoff, a specialist in programming for college students with learning disabilities, has stated, if students take only two or three college preparatory classes per semester, they may not be prepared for a competitive college curriculum that tends to consist of four or five academic courses.

Students typically visit college campuses in the senior year. We believe it is important for students and parents to make informed decisions. They should gather as much information as possible about the services provided at the colleges they are considering and predict which college will best support the student's academic progress. Students will also, of course, need to determine which college atmosphere feels like a "good fit" for them.

The transition process needs to move students from dependence to independence. School personnel, parents, and especially the students themselves have critical roles in this process. School professionals need to replicate, as much as possible, the demands of college in high school and present the students with the wide range of critical skills and strategies mentioned throughout this chapter. Parents need to provide support and guidance, nurturing and mentoring. They can help identify cognitive strengths, encourage involvement in extracurricular activities, stimulate career exploration, provide a good study environment, and foster independence. And students need to master the academic curriculum, learning strategies, independent living skills, and self-advocacy abilities. They need to become self-regulated, self-determined learners—that is, they need to become motivated problem solvers actively engaged in their own learning. They need to be able to set their own goals, take the initiative for implementing these goals, and take responsibility for their own accomplishments and setbacks.

## PROGRAMS

Given the increasing numbers of college students who have learning disabilities, national awareness of this population, legal mandates, and oftentimes financial benefits, more and more programs for college students with learning disabilities are emerging. This academic and social/emotional support is critical if these young adults are to meet the challenges and the range of responsibilities inherent in college life. While many colleges are providing support for students with learning disabilities, the degree and nature of the support varies greatly from campus to campus. If you were to consult a college guide for students who have learning disabilities (and this is a good idea when investigating colleges), you might find support programs designated as "structured" or "coordinated services" or "services," each label denoting the extent to which support is available. A structured program is the most comprehensive.

In determining whether a program is appropriate for you, it is helpful to gather information about instruction, such as the extent and nature of tutoring; related services, such as therapeutic or career counseling; and, of course, the experience and training of staff members. Additional questions might include:

- Are special courses available, such as a study strategies course, a writing course, or a remedial mathematics course?
- Are auxiliary aids available, such as taped textbooks, tape recorders, word processors, or reading machines?
- How are alternative examination arrangements made? What are the options for exam accommodations?
- Is a special orientation provided for students with learning disabilities?

- How many learning disabilities specialists are on staff?
- What is the maximum number of hours of service given to each student each week? Are these services required?
- Are there workshops for college faculty to acquaint them with the nature and needs of students with learning disabilities?

A careful match should be made between the needs of an individual student and the components of a particular program.

A good example of a comprehensive support program is the Higher Education Learning program (HELP), housed in a small liberal arts college in the New York metropolitan area. The HELP program is designed to aid students to become self-determined learners, function effectively in the college classroom, and achieve academic, social, and emotional success in college. The HELP student is expected to develop those competencies needed to lead a responsible, independent, and productive life. HELP offers a range of services, individualized to accommodate the needs of each student. Students assume the same college requirements and enroll in the same courses as their peers without a learning disability, but receive tutoring by a special educator on a regularly scheduled basis.

The HELP program begins with a summer orientation that offers students a series of workshops to help them become more aware of their learning disability and their unique pattern of strengths and weaknesses; develop self-advocacy abilities; highlight the differences between high school and college; and orient them to the college campus. These first meetings are designed to begin to foster those competencies needed to be self-determined adults. Each new HELP student is paired with an upperclass mentor. The mentors, as a group, conduct one of the workshops and then each provides support as needed over the course of the year. At the conclusion of the four-day orientation, students are asked to formulate a tentative list of personal goals and objectives.

Throughout their years in college, HELP students are provided with one-to-one and small group tutorials two to three times per week. Tutoring by special educators, trained and experienced in working with students who have learning disabilities, is the core feature of the program. The exact nature of these tutorials is based on individual need as collaboratively determined by the student and tutor. In tutoring sessions students are guided to develop a repertoire of learning strategies directly applicable to their courses. Some students may use learning strategies to help them construct meaning from history texts. Others may practice note-taking strategies for a philosophy course. And still others may receive help with time management and with advocacy, such as requesting reasonable accommodations and modifications. For some students, tutoring in the use of learning strategies by the special educator is coupled with content-area tutoring by a fellow college student skilled in that subject.

The college offers two specialized credit-bearing courses for HELP students. The first is a learning strategies course available freshman year, covering such topics as organization of time and materials and strategies for note taking from lectures, for constructing meaning from expository text, and for test preparation and test taking. Any student at the college may take this course. The second is a writing course open only to HELP students. It is typically taken during the first semester of the sophomore year, in lieu of the college's writing requirement. Both the content and mechanics of writing are addressed, as students learn to brainstorm, draft, revise, and edit their work with the help of the instructor and peers.

Among the other services available to HELP students are course planning and advising each semester, implemented jointly by a HELP staff member and the professor who is the student's academic adviser. Personal and career counseling as well as internship opportunities are options for all students on campus; and HELP students are strongly encouraged to avail themselves of these services. HELP students meet every six to eight weeks as a group to discuss social, emotional, and academic issues of personal and group concern.

We feel that programs like HELP are very beneficial for enhancing the success of many students who have learning disabilities. The students feel the benefits as well. One student stated: "The program provides a safety net. It gives me security." Another commented, "Knowing I have the program behind me, I feel comfortable enough, secure enough to ask for accommodations and modifications." The greatest challenge of this or any program is to empower students to sustain their commitment to the wide range of college demands. When they manage to do this, as well as to initiate goal setting, establish reasonable priorities, fully engage in the learning task, and take ownership for directing their own learning, then we believe they can be truly successful.

# 12

## Learning Disabilities and Employment

*I work as an accountant. I enjoy my job. I love mathematics and all kinds of analytical thinking. I am dyslexic. I will always be dyslexic. Words on paper will always intimidate me to some degree.*

All adults face the challenges and rewards of employment, home and family, leisure pursuits, community involvement, emotional and physical health, and personal responsibility and relationships. Adults who have learning disabilities must manage these life demands with an added set of problems.

Society expects adults to be self-supporting, to function within a community, and to exhibit appropriate social behavior. Typically, to be self-supporting one must be employed. Employment for most adults spans a long period of time. It may begin with the exit from high school and continue for fifty or more years. While research on the employment of adults who have learning disabilities is sparse, and the findings that are available reflect the heterogeneity of the population, the information reported is unfortunately discouraging. It suggests that individuals with learning disabilities, as a group, show higher rates of unemployment, have jobs of lower status, receive lower pay, and change jobs more frequently than those without learning disabilities. Of course, there are many individuals at all levels of the workforce who do attain professional success. Further, there are well-documented accounts of persons with learning disabilities throughout history who have made significant contributions to society, among the most notable being Einstein, Edison, Churchill, and Rockefeller.

The available data on unemployment vary considerably. One study, conducted in 1989, indicated that only 38 percent of adults who have learning disabilities work full-time. Other research shows numbers ranging from a low of 36 percent to a high of 87 percent. The National Longitudinal Transition Study of Special Education Students, initiated in 1987 and completed in 1994, indicated that youth with learning disabilities who were out of school no more than five years had comparable employment rates to those without disabilities. In contrast, the National Adult Literacy Survey, conducted in the early 1990s and involving adults with learning disabilities of all ages, showed that 39 percent were employed compared with 51 percent of the general population. The employment rate for females who have learning disabilities is significantly lower than that of females in the general population.

The results of research regarding underemployment is more consistent. Most studies reveal that individuals who have learning disabilities, as a group, hold jobs that are considered by the general public to have low status—for example, fast food workers, factory workers, and laborers. It is hardly surprising, then, that large numbers of adults who have learning disabilities report that they are dissatisfied with their jobs and change jobs frequently.

It is important to keep in mind that adults who have learning disabilities who have above average intelligence, come from middle to higher economic backgrounds, and/or have completed postsecondary education, have higher rates of employment, higher job status, and greater job satisfaction than this research indicates. Those who graduate from college are much more likely to hold professional or managerial positions, for example, than those who have only a high school diploma.

What makes success on the job so difficult for some people with learning disabilities? For one thing, persistent problems with reading, writing, and arithmetic can interfere with their work. Many report that they continue to struggle with decoding skills, sight vocabulary, and reading rate. Banking tasks and money management often bring out their troubles with arithmetic. Spelling is frequently reported to be the biggest problem of all.

The level of basic skills that is required in the current job market is expanding to include more abstract abilities. Employers want their workers not only to be proficient in basic skills but also to be able to use these skills effectively and efficiently to solve on-the-job problems. Employers want the people they hire to be able to read for information, to analyze and synthesize the material, and apply the material read to on-the-job situations. They further expect employees to analyze problems, formulate solutions, and communicate that process, in writing, to others. Workplace mathematics, like reading and writing, also requires identification of the problem, analysis, and then the ability to find a solution.

Employers further expect good interpersonal skills. The ability to use technology and information systems is becoming more essential as well. To do all of these things efficiently and effectively, workers must have mastered basic skills and be able to apply thinking skills. They also need personal qualities such as individual responsibility, self-esteem, and self-management. The nature of a learning disability may affect the development of some of these competencies. For example, because of years of struggle and failure, self-esteem may be low and self-monitoring skills may not be functioning effectively.

Employers often do not understand what a learning disability is, thus making it even more difficult for the adults with learning disabilities whom they supervise. Because employers cannot "see" the disability and may have limited knowledge about learning disabilities, they may find it difficult to understand that the problems are real. Therefore, they may fail to provide the necessary accommodations and supportive environment. They may often fail to recognize that, with assistance, workers who have learning disabilities may be tremendous assets to the company.

In a recent interview study, Beth Greenbaum, Steve Graham, and William Scales—educators whose research interests focus on postsecondary experiences of individuals with learning disabilities—reported that a critical barrier for adults who have learning disabilities in the workplace was their own fear of discrimination. These adults, all college graduates, had disclosed their learning disability to professors and other college personnel but were afraid to tell their employers. They feared that revealing their learning disability during the application process might prevent them from being hired and that revealing it after they were hired would lead to prejudice and stigmatization. Their own fears prevented them from requesting appropriate and reasonable workplace accommodations.

Despite on-the-job challenges and the distressing statistics, many adults who have learning disabilities do achieve occupational and professional success, and we believe that number is increasing. By job success we mean keeping a job over a period of time, being satisfied with the job, advancing professionally, and, for some, attaining prominence in a field. What are the variables associated with success? We have spoken of self-determination, the ability and willingness to select and implement choices to control one's life. In order to be self-determined, one must be assertive, think creatively, have pride in oneself, and be able to self-advocate. Understanding one's strengths and weaknesses and accepting oneself are the foundations of self-determination. Unfortunately, many of the competencies associated with self-determination are the very ones with which individuals who have learning disabilities struggle: the ability to plan, to initiate actions to implement a plan, and to respond flexibly to situations. Self-determination is as important for adults making the transition to employment as for those continuing to college.

Other factors, both within the individual (intrinsic) and within the individual's environment (extrinsic), are associated with success. Intrinsic factors include the motivation to succeed, the willingness to work hard and persist at working hard over an extended period of time, and the willingness to sacrifice to achieve one's goals. Supportive family and friends, employers, teachers, and mentors are critical extrinsic forces. They can help solve problems, bolster self-esteem, and provide assurance and encouragement. Notice that these intrinsic and extrinsic variables are similar to those linked with success in college.

In 1992, Paul Gerber, Rick Ginsberg, and Henry B. Reiff, professors and notable researchers, studied professionally successful adults who have learning disabilities, to determine their views of the correlates of success. They interviewed seventy-one adults, with an average age of forty-five, forty-six of whom were considered highly successful and twenty-five moderately successful. Success was determined by income level, type of job held, educational level, attainment of leadership roles, and job satisfaction.

Overall, this group of adults felt that success is an evolutionary process. It does not just happen. A person must want to succeed, be able and willing to set achievable goals, and work hard and persevere toward these goals. Equally important, the person must confront the learning disability and somehow reinterpret or reframe the experience of having a learning disability in a more productive or positive manner. He or she must identify strengths and use them for successful experiences. At the same time, he or she must be aware of but compensate for weaknesses. Many of the people interviewed used the phrase "gain control over my life." Control, in this context, means making conscious decisions to take charge of one's life, and adapting and changing so as to move forward.

To be successful, this group felt, an individual must turn internal factors, such as the desire to succeed and the awareness and acceptance of a learning disability, into actions. External actions, all related to what we might term "adaptability," might include taking conscious steps toward attaining goals, acquiring strategies for learning, selecting an environment that capitalizes on personal strengths, and developing a network of support systems like parents, friends, teachers, and mentors. Again, note that the variables related to success in employment are similar to those correlated with success in college.

## TRANSITION TO EMPLOYMENT

Transition planning is designed to prepare young people to meet the many demands and complexities of adult life, including employment, postsecondary education, community involvement, daily living, health, leisure, and personal and social relationships. For the transition planning process to work, there must be participation and coordination of school programs, adult agency services, and other available supports within the community. Transition planning for those with learning disabilities should begin early, no later than age fourteen. Some aspects of the transition process, such as career exploration, can even begin in elementary school. Students should assume, to the greatest extent possible, responsibility for goal setting, and to do so successfully they need to be taught strategies for decision making. Family members must also be integrally involved in the process, and the needs, values, and situations of the family must be considered as well. Transition planning needs to encompass all facets of adult life.

The need for transition planning for young people who have disabilities has been recognized for the past thirty years. This includes all categories of disabilities. But it was not until 1990 that transition planning was mandated, by law, for all students ages sixteen and older who have disabilities, and this mandate appears as part of IDEA. These federal regulations became effective in November 1992. In the reauthorization of IDEA, in 1997, transition begins to be addressed at age fourteen.

We believe that transition planning for persons who have learning disabilities has lagged behind other groups with disabilities for a number of reasons, three in particular. First, the general public erroneously believes that a learning disability is only a school-related issue, and that individuals with learning disabilities do not encounter problems with employment or other issues related to adult living. Second, traditional transition models were developed for those with more serious disabilities and more limited employment opportunities. And finally, the learning-disabled population is diverse, and planning for such a heterogeneous and complex group, with a broad range of strengths and needs, is more difficult than for other disabled populations. Some students who have learning disabilities may require help with a single domain, like career awareness. Others may need intensive, ongoing support in a number of areas, such as social skills or independent living skills or academics, in addition to career exploration and vocational training.

The educational community is now beginning to address the transition needs of individuals who have learning disabilities. They recognize that a learning disability does not disappear with the completion of school. They are also responding to the emerging research, noted earlier, that shows that the population who has learning disabilities, when viewed as a group, demonstrates greater unemployment, employment in jobs of lower status, and less job satisfaction than those who have no such disabilities. And we have some research—not much, unfortunately, as yet— that suggests that students who have learning disabilities who receive vocational education during high school are more successful in the job market than those who do not. We recognize that vocational education is only one component of a comprehensive transition planning process. Much more research is needed.

A multifaceted team must plan transition. The core player is, of course, the student. The student needs the support of family members who, among other things, can provide meaningful information about the student's functioning, aspirations, and interests. Other critical members might include educators, potential employers who can provide real work training, adult agency personnel, recreation program directors, and community leaders. Ginger Blalock, a professor who has written a great deal about the transition from school to adulthood, emphasizes the importance of a community team. She states that when a transition planning team includes representatives from agencies within the community, and when such members work together, a comprehensive and meaningful continuum of options is developed. Also to be considered are the educational, economic, cultural, and social factors relevant to the particular locale within which the student lives and plans to work. For example, how do the student's goals match the needs of the community, and how can he or she capitalize upon the community's existing job opportunities and educational, social, and cultural activities?

Given the diversity of the population who has learning disabilities, transition programming must not only be comprehensive but individualized, based on personal needs, interests, and preferences. The written individualized transition plan should be the coordinating mechanism for services. It should include a vocational component that covers systematic vocational assessment, career exploration, job training, and vocational counseling to help set realistic goals. Vocational training needs to be diverse enough to reflect the range of occupational roles held by individuals who have learning disabilities.

Indeed, every aspect of transition planning for individuals who have learning disabilities must consider the heterogeneity of the learning disabled population. Some individuals may require job-seeking skills, such as résumé writing, interviewing, and completing job applications, in addition to the vocational competencies listed here. Others may need continued support with academic skills, and the academic skills for employment may be quite different than those required for college. Like transition planning for college, planning for employment needs to help the young adult be aware of his or her own learning disability, accept his or her own strengths and weaknesses, and develop the range of competencies associated with self-determination.

Today, high school students with learning disabilities are fortunate to be able to participate in transition planning. This planning should help them attain success in the workplace. But we believe that adults who have learning disabilities who are currently in the workforce but never received such services can still achieve occupational success. Supportive individuals in their environment like employers, family members, and friends, workplace accommodations, and psychological interventions (see chapter 10) can facilitate their success.

## THE LAW

There are laws that provide opportunities for young adults who have learning disabilities as they prepare for work and others that protect them once they are on the job. We have already discussed the mandate for transition planning contained in IDEA. This mandate is designed for all young adults who receive special education services to prepare them for adult life. There are initiatives, as well, for the general population to develop competencies needed for adult employment, including two school reform programs known as the Tech-Prep Act and School-to-Work Opportunities Act. Students who have learning disabilities can take advantage of these programs as well.

The Tech-Prep Act, passed in 1990 as an amendment to the Perkins Vocational and Applied Technology Education Act, encourages an extensive reorganization of vocational programs to better prepare students for the world of work. Among other provisions, this Act requires that curricula of vocational programs clearly tie academic- and job-related information to the workplace. Curricula are to include such competencies needed in the workplace as basic reading, writing, math, listening, and speaking skills; thinking skills like decision making, problem solving, and reasoning; and personal qualities such as responsibility, self-esteem, sociability, self-management, and integrity. Tech-Prep programs not only offer students a core of academic subjects but also provide opportunities for career planning and for making connections between school and work.

The School-to-Work Opportunities Act, passed in 1994, provides additional opportunities for all students to prepare for the workplace. Through this Act, monies are allocated to states and communities for such programs as Tech-Prep and other school-to-work initiatives. These programs must include a school-based and a work-based learning component, as well as such activities as workplace mentoring, technical assistance for employers, and personal guidance and counseling. Clearly the aim is to provide young adults with opportunities to link classroom education to future employment.

Once on the job, individuals who have learning disabilities are protected under the Vocational Rehabilitation Act of 1973, Sections 503 and 504, and the Americans with Disabilities Act (ADA). To review, Section 503 requires all employers who receive federal contracts or subcontracts to provide reasonable accommodations for qualified individuals with disabilities. Section 504 mandates the same for all facilities, businesses as well as colleges, that receive federal monies.

Since many businesses do not receive federal contracts or monies, most workers with disabilities are protected by the provisions of ADA. ADA was signed into law in 1990. To be protected under ADA, an individual with a disability must be qualified; that is, if provided reasonable accommodations, he or she must be able to perform the essential functions of the job and have the same training and/or experience as would be expected of any other candidate for the job. ADA prohibits discrimination of a qualified individual because of a disability, in areas such as job application procedures, hiring, advancement, discharge, compensation, and job training. There are similarities between ADA and the sections of the Vocational Rehabilitation Act. Both define a disability in much the same way, and both interpret discrimination as a refusal to grant reasonable accommodations for a qualified individual with a disability in the absence of undue hardship.

"Reasonable accommodation" and "undue hardship" are determined on a case-by-case basis. Reasonable accommodations in the workplace might include altering existing facilities to make them more accessible— for example, providing ramps for individuals with physical handicaps; restructuring a job so as to provide flexible scheduling; providing readers or note takers; adjusting examinations—like, for example, providing extended time—or modifying training materials. A reasonable accommodation is one that is deemed sufficient, not necessarily best, to create for the individual an equal employment opportunity. A business need not grant a particular accommodation if it is determined that such an accommodation presents an undue hardship. The nature and cost of the accommodation, the financial resources of the business, and the type of operation and workforce employed are all considered when deciding whether an accommodation is an undue hardship for a business.

For many adults, gainful and productive employment provides the basis of self-esteem and self-fulfillment. It is our hope that, as greater numbers of adults who have learning disabilities benefit from transition planning and programming, receive educational opportunities commensurate with their interests and abilities, and are provided with reasonable accommodations and modifications in school and on the job, more and more will realize their full potential.

# 13

## *Vocational Rehabilitation*

*When I first started my job, the company put me into a training program. This was like a classroom, like going back to school with tests. I needed a certain average on the tests to advance in the company. After I failed the first test, I told the trainer about my learning disability. The remainder of the tests were administered orally, and I did just fine.*

Vocational rehabilitation is a federal and state program designed to assist individuals who have disabilities in obtaining gainful and productive employment that is consistent with their capabilities, interests, resources, priorities, and concerns. The Rehabilitation Services Agency—a federal agency that is a component of the Office of Special Education and Rehabilitation Services, the U.S. Department of Education—has the ultimate responsibility for vocational rehabilitation programs. Each state has a vocational rehabilitation agency as well, which directs services under an approved state plan. The actual provision of services is accomplished through local vocational rehabilitation offices.

## THE LAW

The Rehabilitation Act of 1973 and its subsequent amendments are the governing legislation for the Rehabilitation Services Agency. The purpose of the Act, in this context, is to assist states in operating a vocational rehabilitation system that assesses, plans, and implements services for individuals who have disabilities. The provisions of the Act are designed to empower individuals who have disabilities to maximize their employment potential as well as their economic self-sufficiency and overall independence. The Act ensures that the federal government is actively involved in promoting employment and independent living of individuals who have disabilities.

## VOCATIONAL REHABILITATION AND LEARNING DISABILITIES

Adults who have learning disabilities are the fastest growing disability category served by the vocational rehabilitation system. According to the National Institute on Disability and Rehabilitation Research, the number of learning-disabled adults accessing services rose from 1.3 percent in 1983 to an estimated 5 percent in 1994. Yet adults who have learning disabilities make up only a small percentage of the persons receiving such services. And although more and more adults who have learning disabilities are taking advantage of vocational rehabilitation programs, the number is still significantly smaller than that of high school students who have learning disabilities participating in special education programs.

Why is the number so small? Perhaps special education professionals in the secondary schools lack information about vocational rehabilitation services and therefore cannot appropriately guide students. Perhaps special educators and vocational rehabilitation counselors view learning disabilities as merely an academic, school-related issue, rather than a lifelong problem that can affect one's employment. It was not until 1981 that the Rehabilitation Services Agency included learning disabilities as a recognized category for services. Clearly, all adults who have learning disabilities do not need vocational rehabilitation services. Those who do, have deficits that might substantially impede employment.

Vocational rehabilitation agencies have adopted their own definition and have implemented diagnostic and eligibility criteria for providing services to individuals who have learning disabilities. The definition reads as follows:

A specific learning disability is a disorder in one or more of the central nervous system processes involved in perceiving, understanding and/or using concepts through verbal (spoken or written) language or nonverbal means. This disorder manifests itself with a deficit in one or more of the following areas: attention, reasoning, processing, memory communication, reading, writing, spelling, calculation, coordination, social competence and emotional maturity. [RSA, 1995]

Note that this definition, in contrast to others described in earlier chapters, mentions problems with attention, memory, coordination, social competence, and emotional maturity. Vocational rehabilitation professionals believe these are the problems most closely associated with difficulties with employment. (See also chapter 2 for a review of definitions.)

Berkeley Planning Associates, in 1989, conducted a nationwide study examining vocational rehabilitation services provided to individuals who have learning disabilities and the characteristics of the individuals accessing them. It was found that the average overall IQ of individuals who have learning disabilities using such services is lower than that of the general population of individuals who have learning disabilities. (The average IQ was 86, as compared to 90 or higher.) Also, they tend to have completed fewer years of school—on average, tenth grade is the highest grade completed. Individuals who have learning disabilities tend to use vocational rehabilitation services because they are underemployed rather than unemployed, as is the case with other groups with disabilities. On the average, it costs less to provide services to individuals with learning disabilities than it does to other groups, since they tend to require far fewer services and their long-term outcomes tend to be better.

## THE EVALUATION

Any person can be referred to a vocational rehabilitation agency for services. It is recommended that individuals begin to be involved with vocational rehabilitation offices while in high school, and some states begin to work with people as young as fifteen. After referral, an evaluation is performed to determine eligibility, a decision made by the vocational rehabilitation counselor. The counselor must decide upon eligibility within sixty days after an application is completed.

A vocational rehabilitation counselor conducts an initial interview that begins the assessment process. With the applicant's permission, the counselor will collect data from a variety of sources, including school records, previous testing, and medical history. A comprehensive vocational assessment follows, which focuses on career interests, functional limitations, and capabilities. Data taken from a range of evaluation measures are analyzed within the context of seven competencies: mobility, communication, self-care, self-direction, interpersonal skills, work tolerance, and work skills. The vocational rehabilitation counselor secures information about the individual's academic abilities and intelligence as well as perceptual, language, and behavioral functioning. There is also a situational assessment, in which the individual is observed in a real or simulated job setting. In addition, work attitudes, work habits, work tolerance, and social and behavior patterns are evaluated.

## ELIGIBILITY FOR SERVICES

Most vocational rehabilitation agencies will not automatically accept a school's label of a learning disability as an official diagnosis. The diagnosis must be made by a licensed physician or psychologist trained to identify individuals with learning disabilities, and it must comply with the guidelines specified by the Act and its amendments. The diagnostic battery in schools, typically limited to measures of academic achievement and intelligence, is reportedly not sufficient to provide vocational rehabilitation counselors with information about the impact of learning disabilities on employment potential.

Diagnosis of a learning disability by a qualified professional, however, does not guarantee that a person will be eligible for services. The disability must be severe enough to significantly interfere with one or more of the seven areas of functioning listed by the Act and its amendments. Limitations in one or more of these areas, in turn, impedes employment. In addition, the individual must require multiple vocational rehabilitation services over an extended period of time.

## THE SERVICES

Vocational rehabilitation services are available to eligible persons who are unemployed, at risk of losing their jobs, or underemployed. The focus of all vocational rehabilitation services is on employment. There is no standard package of services. Rather, the vocational rehabilitation counselor works individually with the client to determine career goals and objectives and needed services and accommodations.

Based on information gathered during assessment, the vocational rehabilitation counselor, in consultation with the client, develops an Individualized Written Rehabilitation Plan (IWRP). The primary purpose of this plan is to have individuals achieve employment objectives that match their unique capabilities, interests, and resources. The plan includes items such as long-term goals and short-term objectives, vocational rehabilitation services to be provided, technology services, and related personal assistance services. The individual must state how he or she was involved in choosing goals, objectives, and service providers. IWRP's are updated at least once annually. If appropriate, the vocational rehabilitation counselor, on behalf of the client, accesses community agencies such as a mental health agency, public employment office, or Social Security Administration.

All services are geared toward preparing the individual for employment and keeping him or her employed. For an individual who has a learning disability, critical services might include career counseling and work-related placement assistance that helps with a job search, placement, and job retention. Vocational training might also be helpful, as might technological aids and services. A word about training: the vocational rehabilitation agency will typically not pay for tutoring in higher-education institutions unless there is evidence that maximum efforts have been made to obtain resources elsewhere.

As we have noted earlier, although the number of adults who have learning disabilities using vocational rehabilitation services is ever increasing, services are accessed by only a small percentage of the learning disabled population. For some, whose deficits may impede performance on the job, such services may indeed maximize employment potential. It is our hope that as a greater proportion of the population recognizes that a learning disability is not merely a school issue, vocational rehabilitation services will become more of an option, and vocational rehabilitation professionals, as knowledgeable advocates, will help greater numbers be self-supporting contributors to society.

# 14

## *Interviews with Adults with Learning Disabilities*

The stories in this chapter represent interviews with eight individuals who have learning disabilities. Some we worked with in support programs, and others we saw for evaluation or consultation. Each person has found his or her own way to cope with the disability by "reframing" the problems into positive solutions. The disability has nevertheless played a significant role in each of their lives.

### MICHAEL

Michael is a twenty-five-year-old special education teacher who has just completed a master's degree in elementary and special education. He maintained a solid A average in graduate school. This fall, Michael will be again teaching at a special school for children with learning disabilities.

Michael's father, brother, and sister all have a history of learning disabilities. Michael was first diagnosed at the age of eight, when he was in third grade. He was referred to the school-based committee on special education because of difficulty mastering reading and writing skills. Michael remembers that his silent reading was slow and his oral reading hesitant and labored, with little attention to punctuation and phrasing. He had great difficulty mastering phonic skills, which affected his ability both to decode and to spell. When first told he had a learning disability, Michael reportedly felt confused: "No one really explained what a learning disability was."

Michael received resource-room support services until he graduated from high school. He remembers his greatest difficulty being with reading:

I would read a whole page of text and have little understanding. Reading aloud . . . well, I hated reading aloud because it reflected my trouble with decoding. My writing was variable, as my content was always good but I had trouble with mechanics. I was generally fine with mathematics, although fractions were hard. I never did master fractions. All in all, my first five years in school were torture. During the summer, on the other hand, I was free from the songs that haunted me: "Moron, dummy, what's wrong with you, everyone else can do it, stop acting so stupid."

Michael describes his school experience, overall, as follows:

It was a source of a lot of anger. I was a truly horrible student until sixth grade, when my father died. Something changed for me following my father's death. I wanted to help my family. The only thing I could think of was to take care of my own learning. I wanted to be known as smart. I began to work so hard. And I had help. I had wonderful resource-room teachers who taught me strategies. But most importantly they were very supportive. They made me feel good about myself. I could yell and curse at them, and let out all my frustrations, and they would understand. It was not that I didn't respect them. In fact, I respected them more than anyone. They made me feel safe.

Unfortunately, in the classroom I wasn't always safe. In fact, I remember one incident in junior high school that still sends shivers up my spine. It was the first day of school. I was sitting in my seat in English class suddenly nauseated as each student was called upon to read aloud. My life as I saw it was soon to come to an end. I can't do this. Sweat began to seep through my pores and sizzle upon the surface of my forehead.

I watched as the teacher scanned the room to select a row of readers. As his head spun in my direction, I dropped my pencil on the floor. I have affectionately come to call this the "submarine," one of the evasive tactics in my repertoire. The teacher called my name. I wasn't safe. While I fumbled through the pages, it became apparent to the entire class that I had no idea where we were. "Page 13," the teacher called out, as I continued to search. "We'll come back to you," he said. I was off the hook, but only for the time being. He began again with the front of the row and I knew there would be no getting around this twice. I would have to read.

I could hear the girl three seats ahead of me reading aloud. She read beautifully and, for a second, I forgot the horror of my situation. The words from her mouth flowed softly and gently. She caught every nuance and expressed each emotion. "There's no way that this is the first time she's read this," I thought.

Just then it occurred to me that I could read over the parts that I would be asked to read. I figured that with the two people left between me and the girl who was reading now, I should have just enough time to preread the two pages that would be assigned to me. I skipped ahead and began to practice.

As the person directly in front of me was called upon, I could feel my heart pound at my chest and neck. Continuing to read over what I thought would be my part, I gained in hope and confidence. It was now my turn. I gripped my book tight. "Michael," he bellowed, "skip ahead to page 28. . . ." I lost all feeling in my hands, and the pages slipped through my fingers. This can't be happening. There was nothing left to do but read. I picked the book up, turned to page 28, and began to read.

At first I did all right and, despite a few chuckles at my monotone interpretation, I felt quite proud of myself. As I read on, I decided that I was going to read like my predecessor, who had read with grace and fluidity. However, the harder I tried to read like my peers, the more I sounded as though I belonged back in my first-grade reading group, the Bluejays.

The class laughed and laughed, louder and louder. The teacher yelled. The bell rang. The book fell from my hands. I said nothing. I never returned to that classroom. That night, I cried myself to sleep.

My greatest growth was in high school. The time from sophomore year to senior was like twenty years, not four. And the growth was probably more emotional than academic. I began to see myself as someone who could succeed. I was no longer a failure. I have to give a great deal of credit for this growth to my high school resource-room teacher.

Until high school I hated reading. I really hated it! Then I took a literature course and I read *Appointment in Samara*, by John O'Hara. What a wonderful book! It was the first time I got everything from the text. That is, I recognized all the symbolism. I began to read a lot after that. In fact, I minored in literature in college. I read all the time now. My books are my trophies. I love going to old bookstores and collecting books.

I feel I have come a tremendous way. I try to look at each of my failures as a door of opportunity. But sometimes the struggle and the memory of the struggle creep up on me. I believe the support of teachers and other significant people have contributed most to my success. A lot of small successes and positive feedback had an enormous impact. I now view my life as a continual series of learning experiences. Learning is an adventure, no longer a chore.

I am often hard on myself; I want to do everything perfectly, but I know I can help others celebrate small successes. When I can no longer make others feel good, I will have to find something else to do with my life. I have a few principles to guide my teaching. Teachers need to figure out how children learn. Failure is opportunity. Love is the most important teaching technique. I believe if all teachers adopted such principles, they would preserve the emotional health of the children they teach.

## MARLENE

Marlene is a forty-five-year-old homemaker. She lives with her husband and two teenage daughters in a suburb of New York City. Marlene's father has a learning disability, as do her brothers, children, nieces, and nephews.

Marlene was not evaluated as a child. She discovered she had a learning disability about twelve years ago when her older daughter was diagnosed and labeled: "Finding out I had a learning disability was a relief. Before that, I thought I was just stupid. Learning disabilities wasn't a term when I was growing up."

School was hard for Marlene. Trouble began in first grade, when she had to learn to read and spell. When trying to read, throughout the early years, she would skip words, mix up letters, omit whole lines of text. And phonic decoding was nearly impossible: "Teachers would train us in vowels. I still do not perceive the difference between the sounds of *a, e, i, o,* and *u*. The sounds meant nothing to me; they still don't. I had no idea what they were talking about when they told me to sound out words."

Writing was even harder than reading and made her much more anxious. The content of her writing was fine, but she had trouble with the mechanics. Marlene went to a reading tutor to help her with reading and writing and to a language therapist: "I needed language work because I had some trouble expressing myself. Certain words, like *hippopotamus*, I just couldn't pronounce. I still can't say *ambiguous* without help. It really wasn't an articulation issue, but rather a language difficulty." In contrast to reading and writing problems, Marlene was strong in math:

> The only time I remember feeling exceptional in a positive sense was one day in third grade when I had a math thing to do. It was like a contest; how fast you could complete ten problems. I beat Arnie Rosenberg, the brightest of the bright. The teacher made me do the task three times because she couldn't believe I could beat Arnie. That day I really wondered how I could beat Arnie and, at the same time, not be able to read.

Marlene's social skills were strong as well. She always had a lot of friends, although in school, because of her problems with academics, she often felt somewhat awkward. Outside of school she was very popular.

Throughout junior and senior high, largely because of her very hard work, Marlene achieved average grades. She was accepted to a competitive university. After six months, however, Marlene discovered that it was not right for her. She transferred to a two-year business school in New York City specializing in fashion merchandising, where she ultimately obtained an associate's degree:

> This school had a whole training program that included how to do your hair, your nails, how to maintain your weight. Everything was checked once a week. I did fine with the personal hygiene but, unfortunately, I still had to get through the academic part; that is, writing the papers and reading. We didn't have a word processor, so you can just imagine how my papers looked when I typed them. What a mess! However, I did very well with any task that involved math. A nice smile and good social skills took me a long way. All in all, I was very successful in this school.

Marlene was also very successful in her professional life. Upon graduation from the business school, she was hired by a major corporation and advanced rapidly. In fact, after only three years of employment, she was honored as being one of the most successful graduates of her business school. Marlene traveled all over the world, made presentations at conferences, and moved up the corporate ladder. She was always a hard worker, never found a task too big or too small. She was always willing to help people, who were then more than happy to help her in return. She was ambitious, smart, and personable. And Marlene learned how to circumvent some of her academic problems: "I always hired assistants who could write. They always wrote better than I. But that was okay. I was more creative."

At forty-five, Marlene says she is very happy:

I take care of my family. I play bridge and I love it. I get to use my math skills in bridge, and overall I feel very accomplished. I don't know what I am going to do next in terms of my professional life. But that's okay. I'm content. I feel so lucky that I'm not nervous or anxious about something. I'm enjoying the peacefulness of my life.

I still struggle with reading and writing issues, of course. I rarely read. I can fall asleep after reading only five pages. And I read very slowly. I'd much rather read a brochure than a book. If I go to the library, I do so to rent videos. Maybe when I am much older and have lots and lots of time with nothing to do, I'll go to the library to borrow a book. If I have to read, I do, of course, but I really need to know something about the subject to get the meaning. The more I know about the subject and the greater my interest, the better my reading. Sometimes, if the vocabulary is unfamiliar, I feel as if I am dealing with a foreign language.

Writing was and is very difficult. And writing makes me very nervous; much more so than reading. If I read, I don't have to read aloud anymore. But when writing, I need to put my thoughts on paper. It's out there from me to you. It's there to be judged.

Reflecting upon my life and my own struggles, I would say to others just beginning to address their learning disability, never give up. You don't have to be the best at everything. But learn about yourself. Discover your own strengths and weaknesses. Find the area you are good at and pursue it. Work on the good stuff.

## JANE

Jane is a fifty-five-year-old school nurse who has taught health education in a public school for the last ten years. She lives with her husband and son in New York City. She was trained as a registered nurse in France, but left the field for a brief time in order to complete a degree in art history. Now she is back in nursing, enjoying her work in a school, teaching and caring for her students.

There is a strong family history of learning disabilities, which is traced to her mother's side. Jane's grandfather, two of his children, Jane herself, her sister, a nephew, as well as several cousins all have some type of learning disability. Jane was first evaluated when she was eight years old. At that time the diagnosis was "word blindness." Since few people knew of this, Jane's mother read all that was available, so that she could help Jane's teachers understand her problems.

Jane describes her school experience as "horrible." She found it hard to learn to read or spell and as a result felt frustrated most of the time. She remembers that her one wish was to "get rid of it."

Jane attributes some of her problems to the fact that she read slowly, as "words and letters seemed to jump around." She read the beginning of a word, but guessed the end. She describes her comprehension as "okay, not great." It was hampered by the fact that she read slowly, and made many decoding errors. By the time she got to the end of the passage, she found she had lost the meaning. Even at this point she finds reading to be laborious. Her attention is variable, and in order to fully understand the material, she has to reread passages two to three times. While Jane does enjoy novels, she avoids lengthy technical material.

The content and organization of Jane's writing have always been good, and she has done well in mathematics. But she remembers being unable to spell. Throughout high school, teachers "harassed and humiliated" her when she could not spell in front of the class, and she was even penalized for spelling errors on written assignments and tests, which of course depressed her grades.

Jane received intermittent help, first in a Child Guidance Center and then with a friend of her mother. But she did not find this support helpful, as "strategies were never taught." While her mother always served as her advocate and understood the nature of her disability, she was still unable to accept Jane's problems: "She always treated me as if I were damaged." Jane also had to cope with the fact that almost all the members of her family were college graduates. Some were even professors. In high school, Jane remembers feeling exceptionally proud when she passed several advanced courses, finally proving to her family that she was "as smart" as her sister.

Jane now has many friends and is successful in her work and marriage. But she feels that the learning disability had a "powerful effect" on her life. She was shy and insecure as a child and still does not feel confident. While successful, she feels that the disability colored her sense of herself and therefore her ability to pursue both academic and professional goals.

As a nurse, she is particularly careful about rereading medical orders for children in her school. She has problems entering data and tends to reverse the numerals in telephone numbers, but she is alert to these problems and able to self-correct. Jane describes herself as "creative, task-oriented, and good at mediating and negotiating for others." These skills have certainly helped her at each stage of her life. Jane still thinks about getting help, particularly with reading, but she feels it may be too late. "I would do something if I thought it would help." She continues: "My heart bleeds, though, for other kids who struggle with a learning disability. . . . They should get help as soon as possible."

## STEVE

Steve is a twenty-nine-year-old graduate student. He has two master's degrees in education and is now completing his doctorate in educational administration. He is working on his dissertation and hopes to complete his degree within the next two years. His goals are to look for a job that will allow him to teach, work with administrators and teachers, and write fiction as well as books about education.

While there is no documented family history of learning disabilities, Steve remembers that his mother often missequenced letters, and he heard stories that his grandmother, a respected physician, also may have had some learning problems. Steve was first diagnosed in second grade. While his parents explained to him that he learned differently and more slowly than others, he interpreted this to mean that his "brain didn't work right."

Once he was diagnosed, his parents moved him from a public to a private school, where he had to repeat second grade. He was initially devastated by this change, not wanting to leave his friends. On his first day at the new school, he was called to the blackboard to interpret an array of mathematical problems. Without a context, he remembers having no idea what he was being asked to do:

> In third grade, I was frustrated and angry and so became very unruly in school. In fourth grade, my teacher insisted that I use a typewriter in the classroom because she couldn't read my handwriting. But I did not want to seem different. My father respected my feelings and convinced the teacher to give up this plan. Toward the end of the year, I was introduced to the computer, and by middle school I was able to do basic programming.

During the early grades, Steve had an overriding sense of being lost and not being as good as the others. In fact, he remembers having difficulty relating to other children: "I had low self-esteem, could not keep up with my friends, and was always a little at odds with the group. My classmates preferred to play with my [older] brother than with me."

Steve was always good at writing and felt more comfortable communicating on a written than a verbal level. Math and science were his weakest subjects: "Math was unbelievable . . . couldn't do it." Steve also describes the fact that he had significant memory problems: "If I was told to do things, twelve seconds later, all the directions were gone. I couldn't follow the steps to complete a task."

In sixth grade, he achieved an A in Latin, and by ninth grade he was able to manage A's and B's in most subjects. From tenth through twelfth grades, he attended an all-boys' school: "While these years were generally awful, I did manage to pass. However, even though I was a good reader, I had difficulty getting the concepts in courses such as, Modern European History."

Steve was tutored in his academic subjects until he started high school, which greatly improved his skills. He also met with a child psychiatrist with whom he was able to "talk about things." In fact he remembers this as the "biggest help . . . being able to talk about ongoing issues and go over questions on a day-to-day basis."

Steve applied to a small liberal arts college and was accepted as an early admission. Although the first year was a little chaotic, he did not need remedial help. He continued to have problems with mathematics, and so withdrew from Statistics. "I liked college; I was motivated. I got interested in things. I had ideas people thought were good."

After college, Steve completed a series of literature courses in order to qualify for a doctoral program in English. But he was rejected in two application rounds from ten schools. He decided to teach and was able to find a job at an elementary school. He soon realized he loved the work. After several years of teaching, he applied for a graduate degre in education and was accepted to a competitive program, where he has done exceptionally well. He feels at ease with the work, although statistics and research design continue to be difficult for him.

In thinking back to the help Steve received as a child, he clearly identifies his father as amost significant person: "My father was open and always seemed to understand. He always put things in perspective and pointed out the gains I made." Steve recalls an early stormy relationship, though, with his brother, who was two years older, and a "neatly organized, superstar in school". Until ninth or tenth grade, his brother never called him by his name but referred to him as "Retardo." Steve and his brother are now friends.

Steve describes his learning disability this way:

> I can do two things at once, but am better at doing one at a time. . . . My room is a mess, papers, books flying everywhere, and you would not want to see me organize a meal. My social skills are fine, although I tend to compete with my friends. I guess that's because I never had a chance to shine when I was young. I always felt inferior; my friends beat me in everything.

Now, Steve likes his work and feels that becoming a teacher is the best thing that happened to him. He believes strongly that children who have learning disabilities should have the opportunity to talk openly with parents and other adults and not be embarrassed. Otherwise, frustration can build up.

## TIMOTHY

Dr. Timothy Frank is a fifty-year-old obstetrician who has a learning disability. Timothy was evaluated as an adult after his son was diagnosed: "I realized I had a learning disability when I sat at the parent conference for my son and the professionals described his problems to me. I recognized that they were very much the same problems I had and still have. What I regret is that I didn't know about my problems earlier. I might have had a lot more success at school."

While he was in school, at least for the early years, it was thought that Timothy was just not bright or perhaps that he wasn't trying. His first vivid memory of a problem was in second grade, when he just could not seem to grasp the addition of two-digit numbers. Math was always Timothy's area of significant difficulty.

Although he tried hard in school, he seemed unable to get good grades and his self-esteem suffered: "I felt dumb, dumb, dumb, as I tried, failed, and the kids made fun of me." As he lost confidence in himself, his performance in other school subjects began to falter as well. Timothy's social skills were intact, but because of his poor grades he was often teased and felt awkward around his peers. He was the last to be chosen for games and often felt left out.

From the time he was seven years old, Timothy knew he wanted to be a doctor. As school became harder and harder, medical school seemed like an unrealistic dream. He loved science, but then had a great deal of difficulty with chemistry and physics in high school, largely due to his problems with mathematics. School counselors told him that without good grades in these two subjects, medical school would not be an option. He spent many summers in school, redoing math courses and working very, very hard at the sciences. Failed tests, hours and hours of tutoring, and tremendous effort are what Timothy largely remembers about high school: "If my classmate took an hour to complete an assignment, I would have to take two and sometimes three."

Because of his perseverance, stubbornness, enormous effort, innate strength, and refusal to accept defeat, Timothy made his way through high school and college and was ultimately accepted to medical school:

I had to work very hard to get by. I think because I had to put in so much effort, I learned to work hard even in areas that were not particularly difficult for me. My tremendous drive seemed to spill over onto everything. I think this caused me to be a much better student than some others for whom schoolwork was much easier.

Timothy says he finds being an adult with a learning disability far less a problem than being a child with a one. He does not have to study mathematics or chemistry or prove himself through exams. He is a fine physician, and his problems have little impact on his day-to-day work.As a child, he remembers, he had real questions about whether he could be successful in life. And his self-esteem was low. As an adult, he shares his experiences with his children, who struggle with much the same issues he did more than forty years ago.


## SAM

Sam is a fifty-seven-year-old physician. He has held a responsible position in a teaching hospital for over twenty years. He maintains a private practice and is regarded as a caring and gifted doctor.

Sam is the only member of his family who has a learning disability. He was never identified or evaluated, but he always knew he had problems.

In thinking about his school years, Sam describes himself as a "bad student." Learning problems were most evident in the early grades, where he had trouble with phonics and spelling. He did not learn the alphabet until third grade—which came as a surprise to his parents, who apparently did not notice the delay. To them, he seemed to be functioning quite well in every way. Sam's reading was slow and labored. When he had to say and spell a word in front of the class, he could not even retain the word long enough to spell it. Sam remembers feeling ashamed and embarrassed.

Fortunately, Sam's reading comprehension has always been a strength, as is his reading vocabulary. His oral vocabulary is not as strong. He describes himself as "talented" in mathematics, logic, and problem solving, and it was these skills that helped him understand the logic of an essay or the content of classroom material. By age twelve or thirteen, he was at the top of his class.

Sam graduated from a competitive college and medical school. But the first two years of medical school were a struggle, as the demands moved from logic to memorization of facts. Sam always had difficulty recalling specific information, such as names, and he mispronounces words when speaking. These problems with oral language are extremely painful for him. He is sure that he has been the "butt of jokes," and so takes care to choose his words carefully to avoid errors.

While Sam struggled with these problems, he never thought of them as symptoms of a learning disability. Only when he was in psychotherapy (in medical school) did it all make sense. This time was particularly important for him, as he gradually gained insight and came to terms with his difficulties. He feels that his therapist helped him make connections while providing the support and help he needed during this time of discovery.

## BARBARA

Barbara is a twenty-six-year-old head teacher in a preschool for children with special needs. She is completing her master's degree in early childhood special education. After completing the degree, she still hopes to keep her job, as she enjoys working with the children and supervising staff. Her long-term goal is to complete a doctorate in developmental psychology. Barbara also works in a bookstore, where she is responsible for the children's story hour.

Barbara is the only member of her family with a learning disability. While she does not remember having difficulty with reading comprehension, she did have problems with phonics, particularly the short and long vowels, and with spelling: "I flunked spelling in first grade even though I sat up at night trying to memorize the words. I hated first grade with a passion. The teacher was mean and I got yelled at when reading aloud." While Barbara made many decoding errors, she had a good sight vocabulary and was able to use context clues to get meaning: "I knew what it meant, and could paraphrase stuff." As for her writing, it "was weak and all jumbled up. I had no concept of structure, couldn't organize my ideas, and my spelling was terrible. My notebooks were a mess, with homework written on scrap pieces of paper. In math, I could never keep the numbers straight and would attack number problems in the middle and add the wrong column."

Barbara was evaluated at age ten, when in fourth grade. But she never quite understood the reason she was having so many problems. As a follow-up to the recommendation, she was tutored from the fourth through the seventh grade. She considers this to have been a very special and supportive experience. The tutor gave her confidence and helped her to see that writing is telling a story: "I would speak to myself and write it down or use a tape recorder." She also learned to see a draft as a work in progress, which encouraged her to edit and self-correct.

In high school, Barbara was able to take honors classes. She got good grades and entered a highly competitive college, which was "hell" the first two years: "But, after flunking some courses, I learned fast. I copied my friends' study habits, and followed their timelines. And the computer was a great help." Barbara majored in sociology, and by her senior year she was an A student. But the erratic record, which she attributes to the learning disability, made it difficult for her to get into a graduate program.

Looking back on her school years, Barbara attributes much of her success to the fact that she always had a lot of self-esteem. She felt smart in spite of her problems, and she believes that her mother's support made this happen. Her mother always told her, "You are smart enough to do anything, if you try and work hard." While Barbara is happy in her work, she acknowledges that the learning disability continues to play a significant role in her life. "The learning disability makes it hard to do things that shouldn't be hard to do, like writing coherently, and speaking a foreign language."

As we can see, a learning disability may look different in each person, and each individual's struggle to overcome his or her problems is poignant. These stories highlight the fact that the disability affects one's social and work performance. But, through adaptive work and application, individuals who have learning disabilities can and do achieve success and reach personal goals.

# 15
## *Conclusion*

*A civilization can be measured by the meaning
which it gives to the full cycle of life. . . . Psychosocial
strength . . . depends on a total process which regulates
individual life cycles, the sequence of generations, and
the structure of society simultaneously: for all three
have evolved together.*
                                                —Erik H. Erikson

A learning disability is a lifelong condition. Some adults, by the time they have completed their formal education, have learned to compensate for their difficulties. For many others, difficulties continue and to varying degrees impact on careers, social relationships, and activities of daily living. There are adults who were diagnosed as children and received services under the guidelines of PL 94-142. But more and more adults, who never knew why school was so hard, are now addressing the problem by initiating an assessment and seeking services to help them cope with their disabilities.

Adults who have learning disabilities are a heterogeneous group. Some struggle with reading and writing, some with mathematical tasks, some with the basic challenges of daily life. There are adults who have learning disabilities who have trouble finding and keeping a job; others are professionally successful yet cannot seem to develop a satisfying social life. And there are those who seem to have few problems as they successfully negotiate the range of life's demands.

Adults who have learning disabilities are not merely children with learning disabilities grown up. The impact of having a learning disability differs at each stage of development. And adulthood itself has many stages, each with its unique challenges. Satisfaction or dissatisfaction at one stage does not guarantee the same degree of adjustment at another. At one point, the adult might deal with self-identity, at another with employment and economic independence, and still another with personal responsibility and relationships.

As a group, adults who have learning disabilities represent a broad spectrum of the population. We see individuals of different ages, from different socioeconomic, ethnic, and cultural groups. We see different clusters of social and learning problems that affect education, social, personal, and occupational adjustments.

The field now recognizes the unique needs of the adult who has learning disabilities, and as such has responded by providing legal protection, programs, services, and an ever-developing information base. Where do we stand today?

## THE FIELD TODAY

The field of learning disabilities has traditionally been child-centered and dominated by research, assessment, and intervention approaches and guidelines appropriate for school-age children. In the last ten to fifteen years, however, more attention has been paid to the varied and complex needs of the adult. But it is just a beginning. We as professionals need to continue our work in order to refine our understanding of the wide range of issues related to the adult and, in so doing, better serve adults of all ages.

The field of learning disabilities is very different today from the way it was in the 1960s, when the term learning disability was first introduced. At that time, special education was a state and local responsibility, and special services were available primarily to those who had sensory impairments or significant emotional problems or limited intellectual capabilities. Few supports existed for children who could not learn to read, write, or do mathematics despite high intelligence and adequate schooling. Thus it is not surprising that many of the adults with whom we speak, particularly those older than forty, were sitting in classrooms unable to master the reading and writing curriculum and not knowing why. These adults were not assessed as children, received no support services, and erroneously attributed their failing grades to their own limited intelligence or lack of effort.

Younger adults might have had the opportunity to benefit from the mandates of PL 94-142 and its subsequent amendments. If they were fortunate to have knowledgeable teachers and informed parents, they might have been referred for an assessment, diagnosed, and labeled, and might have received a free appropriate education in the least restrictive environment. Based on individual need, they could have received resource-room support or placement in a special class or special school. And a large number of adults did indeed benefit from support services. We have spoken to many adults who express their gratitude to the special education professionals who taught them the skills and strategies they needed to compensate for their disabilities. Unfortunately, despite the protections of PL 94-142, there are those who have learning disabilities who went undiagnosed and underserved.

Overall, the field of learning disabilities has come a long way. Prior to 1973, there was no Section 504 (of the Vocational Rehabilitation Act) to prohibit discrimination of individuals with disabilities in facilities that receive federal monies. Prior to 1975, there were no guarantees that children and adolescents with learning disabilities would receive a quality education. Prior to 1990, there was no mandate for services designed to help young adults make the transition to postsecondary school or to the world of work. And prior to 1990, there was no legal assurance that workers with learning disabilities would be granted reasonable accommodations and modifications in their place of employment (whether or not their place of employment received federal monies).

Today, many more services are available for adults who have learning disabilities than there were in the 1960s. Transition services exist in high schools, and support programs are emerging on college campuses across the country as the number of students who have learning disabilities attending college and graduate schools continues to rise. While the nature of these programs varies from school to school, many offer tutoring by special educators in study strategies as well as in reading, writing, and mathematical skills.

For those adults who have learning disabilities who do not pursue postsecondary education, a range of program options offers basic skills remediation in reading, writing, and mathematics, as well as instruction in using strategies for problem solving, time management, and reading and writing. Today, adults can learn skills and strategies in a number of settings. They can work with a private tutor—that is, a learning disabilities specialist—or they can enroll in basic education or literacy programs that have been established within the workplace and within agencies and organizations such as libraries, clinics, government departments, secondary schools, and voluntary literacy organizations.

In 1981 the Rehabilitation Services Agency, which oversees vocational rehabilitation programs, first included learning disabilities as a recognized category for services. This was an important step toward extending services and helping individuals with learning disabilities find and keep gainful and productive jobs. Some of these services include career counseling, job placement assistance, vocational training, and the use of technological aids. Today learning disabilities is the fastest-growing disability category served by the vocational rehabilitation system. According to the National Institute on Disability and Rehabilitation Research, the number of adults with learning disabilities who accessed services rose from 1.3 percent in 1983 to an estimated 7 percent in 1994. In spite of this overall increase, the number served represents only a small percentage of the population that has a learning disability. Unfortunately, this is partly due to the fact that many individuals who have learning disabilities are still unaware that these services exist.

Advances in technology since the 1960s have been dramatic. Studies on brain-behavior relationships report that learning disabilities are due to a central nervous system dysfunction. This dysfunction, in turn, interferes with the processing of information on all levels.

The field of learning disabilities has progressed significantly since the 1960s, but there remains much to be done to fully address the needs of adults who have learning disabilities.

## GOALS AND NEEDS

Throughout this book, we have reviewed relevant research findings and have pointed out areas where continued support is needed. Research cannot exist without funding, which comes primarily from government sources, although private foundations also support investigative efforts. Federal public policy is needed to provide direction at the federal, state, and local levels.

The National Institute of Child Health and Human Development, one of sixteen institutes within the National Institutes of Health, has been committed to the study of learning disabilities since 1963. Reportedly, the money it spent on research in learning disabilities and reading disorders grew from $1.75 million in 1975 (this coincided with the passage of PL 94-142) to $11 million in 1990. Yet Barbara Keogh, a psychologist at the University of California, points out that in 1994, only 1 percent of funding from the Department of Education went to research on learning disabilities, in spite of the fact that learning disabilities is the largest special education category.

In 1985, the Health Research Extension Act (PL 99-158) was passed, mandating the development of an Interagency Committee on Learning Disabilities. Its purpose is to encourage the identification of research priorities and review results of studies on learning disabilities. It accomplishes this through five program projects and three learning disability research centers that work on etiology, definition, diagnosis, and comorbidity.

In 1992, a working conference was sponsored through the National Institutes of Health to bring together researchers and clinicians in the different disciplines to talk about definition, diagnosis, and treatment of learning disabilities. While the focus of the conference was primarily on children, much of the data is applicable to the adult. In 1994, a summit on learning disabilities was organized by the National Center for Learning Disabilities. The goals were to encourage the federal government to increase policy initiatives for both children and adults and include learning disabilities on the national agenda. While not exhaustive, these examples do provide evidence of the collaborative work that is going on in the field. And this collaboration is needed, particularly at the federal level, to define, implement, and accomplish goals.

Research in the neurosciences is taking place within medical schools and universities. And this research provides us with a wealth of studies. There is work on brain-behavior relationships and focal areas that affect learning. Studies are pinpointing specific genes that are associated with dyslexia and attention-deficit/hyperactivity disorder, and family clustering studies have identified familial patterns. Other work is focusing or comorbid conditions associated with a learning disability and the effr and benefit of medication on attention-deficit/hyperactivity diso·

Some studies are examining sociocultural variables, psychosocial issues, and the risk and protective factors that affect learning. These factors help us understand what makes some individuals resilient and able to succeed in spite of the disability. Work on executive function and strategy use has already had an impact on the assessment process and is being applied in instructional programs.

At least 80 percent of individuals who have learning disabilities have significant problems with reading and writing. Over the past twenty years, we have largely moved away from the explanation that these problems are due to faulty visual perception of letters and words. Recent research has now identified a strong link between phonological processing—that is, the processing of sounds—and the ability to read and write.

Other work in the field is addressing the need for a more effective operational definition of learning disabilities, a broader and more dynamic approach to testing, and a wider array of tests for the adult. Current definitions do not provide a uniform set of characteristics or define subgroups. And since we know that the disability looks different in children and adults, we must look toward developing a definition that specifically describes the behavior of adults with learning disabilities.

While the traditional assessment consists primarily of standardized tests, many in the field are recommending the use of dynamic approaches that incorporate what we know about learning and metacognition. These approaches look at an individual's approach to learning a task, use of strategies, and ability to benefit from instruction. While the assessment provides recommendations for instructional planning, in many ways our hands have been tied because we have not had a range of materials or well-defined approaches to use with adults. Instead, we have had to rely on upward extensions of material developed for school-age children.

The information gathered from research is integrated into instructional approaches, but continued work is needed on outcome studies. We need to look at the varied instructional approaches and study the effect they have on individuals with different learning needs. We must know what works best and how to measure change at different points in time. Variables—such as curriculum, approach, frequency, and duration of the intervention—must be studied. And, most important, we must be skilled determining whether change is transferred to real-life contexts—in ool, at work, or at home.

We have seen changes in secondary-school programs. For example, individuals with learning disabilities (like all students with disabilities) now benefit from services that promote the transition to postsecondary educational settings or the world of work. Until recently, the predominant focus of transition services was on students with moderate or severe disabilities. This was due largely to the assumption that students with mild disabilities, such as learning disabilities, could move from secondary school to postsecondary school or employment with relative ease. And the services that were available for students with learning disabilities were geared to academic remediation, with little attention to social skill acquisition, independent living skills, career awareness, and vocational training. We now know that many individuals who have learning disabilities need to develop these competencies.

In providing transition services, consideration must be given to the wide range of abilities and disabilities in the heterogeneous group of students labeled learning disabled. For example, while some students may continue onto college, others will enter the workforce, and still others may pursue technical or vocational training. The transition needs of each of these groups of students are, of course, very different. Also, the student who has learning disabilities needs to participate in his or her own transition planning, determine his or her own realistic goals for the future based on informed decision making, and work with professionals to implement these goals.

It is estimated that 3 to 10 percent of adults in this country have learning disabilities. And while many of these individuals have succeeded in postsecondary educational settings and employment, a large number have not achieved a level of literacy needed to function effectively within society. These low levels of literacy interfere with employment opportunities, educational goals, self-esteem, and empowerment. Reports indicate that well over 50 percent of adults who have learning disabilities are involved in adult literacy, basic education, and job-training programs. In fact, it is suggested that these adults are the largest subgroup in these programs. This should alert us to the fact that significant numbers of adults with learning disabilities do not receive appropriate services. They require intervention that is specific to their needs.

While the goal of literacy programs has traditionally been to develop basic skills, programs are now looking to include more advanced reading, writing, mathematical, and technological skills. Many problems continue to interfere with the effectiveness of these programs, however. Not enough research is directed at differentiating subgroups of adults with and without learning disabilities. The lack of an operational definition also interferes with identification and assessment. As a rule, volunteers and professionals have not been trained to work with individuals who have learning disabilities. Thus, they do not fully understand the problems associated with the disability and are hampered in their efforts to provide appropriate services.

Many suggest that collaborative efforts are needed between professionals involved in the adult literacy programs and those involved in the field of learning disabilities. And some suggest that literacy programs should be developed that specialize in the adult who has learning disabilities. While the field has come a long way, there are still significant numbers of adults who have learning disabilities who are struggling to attain basic levels of literacy.

The National Institute for Literacy, established through the National Literacy Act, is assisting federal agencies in order to help them achieve Goal 6 of Goals 2000 (1994). Goals 2000 are eight national education goals to be reached by the year 2000. The Goals 2000: Educate America Act (1994) sets these goals into law. The purpose of the Act is to establish higher academic standards within American schools and to support states and communities in attaining these standards. Goal 6 states that every adult in America will be literate by the year 2000 and able to compete in a global market.

This is a monumental task to accomplish. Illiteracy extends across all ages and groups. But to address the needs of the adult who has learning disabilities, appropriate assessment and intervention approaches must be developed and available. And professionals working with individuals who have learning disabilities must be trained and skilled.

## FUTURE DIRECTIONS

What does the future of the field look like? Research will continue to provide us with new insights concerning learning disabilities and conditions associated with learning disabilities. We will develop better methods and tools to assess and treat the wide range of problems seen in the adult who has learning disabilities.

But federal initiatives will continue to be needed to stimulate and encourage legislation and research. Federal funding will be needed to help improve professional training in teacher education programs and to develop better assessment tools and intervention techniques.

We will reach out more effectively to educate the public at large as well as the population of adults who have learning disabilities. To improve equal access and positive changes in the workplace, in the school, and within the home, the public must be knowledgeable and aware of the fact that we are dealing with a real, although not always visible, disability.

We must help adults who have learning disabilities become successful in today's economy. The literature describes successful adults as those who are proactive and take control. These qualities lead to self-satisfaction and empowerment. History provides us with an interesting example of how empowerment can be effective in a group process. In the 1960s, the early years of the field, public agencies were concerned solely with the needs of children who have learning disabilities. Little or no planning was done for these children when they were to become adults. Indeed, as these children matured and tried to gain access to post-secondary education, rehabilitation, and employment, it became apparent that the systems in place were just not adequate. To a large degree, it was through the efforts of empowered adults with learning disabilities organized into self-help groups that appropriate services became more available in the 1970s. And it was through the work of adults with learning disabilities in the 1980s and 1990s, in collaboration with parent and professional organizations, that private, nonprofit groups became involved in increasing public awareness to the needs of adults with learning disabilities.

This example aptly demonstrates that while a learning disability is a lifelong condition, more and more adults are achieving significant levels of success. This success is evident along personal lines as well as in school or work areas. As we have pointed out, success is strongly dependent on the ability and willingness to work hard, persevere, and reframe the experience of having a learning disability in a more positive manner.

This means being proactive and using the available support systems and interventions that help one learn new and better ways to compensate for the disability. Clearly both internal factors and these external supports are needed to equip adults and help them negotiate in our fast-moving, ever-changing, highly technological society.

# Appendix A

## *Legislation and Court Cases Pertaining to Learning Disabilities*

The following provides a review of the major legislation that protects the rights of children and adults who have learning disabilities.

## LEGISLATION

### Individuals with Disabilities Education Act

The Education for All Handicapped Children Act, Public Law 94-142, passed in 1975, is landmark legislation for children and youth who have disabilities. The first law to include a definition of learning disabilities, it mandated the development of services within the public schools for youngsters with any disability. The law was modified and reauthorized in 1990, at which time it was renamed the Individuals with Disabilities Education Act (IDEA, Public Law 104-476). It was reauthorized again in 1997.

IDEA mandates free, appropriate education in the least restrictive environment for children and youth, ages three to twenty-one. Other critical features include: referral and assessment procedures, procedural safeguards, and guidelines for individualized educational programming. In the 1990 reauthorization, a mandate was added for transition services and plans.

### Rehabilitation Act and Rehabilitation Act Amendments

The Rehabilitation Act (1973) is considered the most significant piece of legislation that protects the civil rights of individuals who have disabilities of all ages. Section 503 of the act requires all employers who receive federal contracts or subcontracts to provide reasonable accommodations for qualified individuals who have disabilities. Section 504 prohibits discrimination of individuals who have disabilities by the federal government and every entity that receives federal monies and assistance or that does business with the federal government. This would include the majority of colleges and universities. In 1974, the act was amended to provide protection to handicapped students in federally supported public schools. In 1987, an amendment (Civil Rights Restoration Act, Public Law 100-259) was passed stating that if any part of a program or activity receives federal financial assistance, then all operations of the program are subject to Section 504.

Section 504 is not age-restrictive and includes nondiscrimination, free appropriate public education, and protection in employment, postsecondary education, and training programs. "Nondiscrimination" includes both physical and program accessibilty.

Congress amended Section 504 (Rehabilitation Act Amendments, Section 506) to ensure greater uniformity with Title I of the Americans with Disabilities Act (ADA). The amendment states that any institution subject to Section 504 will have its conduct measured by the "standards" of Title I of the ADA.

## Americans with Disabilities Act

The Americans with Disabilities Act (ADA, 1990) extends Section 504 by providing standards that prohibit discrimination in *all* programs, services, buildings, and facilities available to the public, including those that do not receive federal funds. This affects both schools and workplaces. Title II of the Act governs public higher education institutions, and applies to state and local governments. Title III governs private higher-education institutions, as they are "places of public accommodation." The regulations outline the provision of services. These include cost, type of service, and accommodations. ADA also uses a broad definition of disability.

ADA states, however, that a business or institution does not have to provide an accommodation if such an accommodation imposes an undue hardship. Hardship is determined by the type and cost of the accommodation, the financial resources of the business or institution, the type of program, and the impact of the accommodation on the program or operation. Both financial and administrative hardship must be evaluated relative to an individual's ability to function effectively and to the parameters of the program or operation.

## Carl D. Perkins Vocational and Applied Technology Act

The Carl D. Perkins Vocational and Applied Technology Education Act Amendments (Public Law 101-392, 1990) update the Carl D. Perkins Vocational Technical Education Act (Public Law 98-524, 1984). This law provides access to "quality vocational educational programs" and mandates that secondary and postsecondary programs are responsible for providing transitional services and for assisting individuals with special needs with applications and accessibility to programs of study and employment. This Act provides the local educational agency (LEA) with the power to decide how the monies will be distributed among the different special populations and includes a formula, based on poverty level, that allows for distribution of basic grant funds according to the greatest need.

## Tech-Prep Act

The Tech-Prep Act, passed in 1990, an amendment of the Perkins Vocational and Applied Technology Education Act, encourages an extensive reorganization of vocational programs to better prepare students for the world of work. It also requires that vocational programs integrate academic and job-related information to be used in the workplace. Curriculums focus on competencies needed in the workplace, such as basic reading, writing, mathematics, listening, and speaking skills; thinking skills, like decision making, problem solving, and reasoning; and personal qualities, such as responsibility, self-esteem, sociability, self-management, and integrity. Tech-Prep programs not only offer students a core of academic subjects, but also provide opportunities for career planning and for making connections between school and work.

## School-to-Work Opportunities Act

The School-to-Work Opportunities Act, passed in 1994, provides additional opportunities for all students to prepare for the workplace. It allocates monies to states and communities for Tech-Prep and other school-to-work initiatives. These programs must include a school-based and a work-based learning component, as well as workplace mentoring, technical assistance for employers, and personal guidance and counseling. The aim is to provide young adults with opportunities to link classroom education to future employment.

## Technology-Related Assistance for Individuals with Disabilities Act Amendments

The Technology-Related Assistance for Individuals with Disabilities Act Amendments ("Tech Act," 1994) replaced the Technology-Related Assistance for Individuals with Disabilities Act (Public Law 100-407, 1988). The three main purposes of the Tech Act are to provide discretionary grants to states to assist them in developing and implementing (1) consumer-responsive, comprehensive, statewide programs of technology-related assistance for individuals with disabilities of all ages; (2) programs of national significance related to assistive technology; and (3) alternative financing mechanisms to allow individuals with disabilities to purchase assistive technology devices and services.

# LITIGATION, OR CASE LAW

The courts are used to interpret and clarify laws, statutes, and regulations. Class action suits brought by groups of individuals or cases brought by individuals who have learning disabilities focus primarily on education and employment. Those concerning education deal with issues of academic accommodations, such as course substitutions, alterations in program of study, and testing accommodations. Other cases deal with the ability of individuals with handicapping conditions to perform in a program or job or with undue hardship on an institution regarding the provision of reasonable accommodations. Cases on employment deal with the impact of the disability on job function, testing, entry examinations, and job accommodations.

The following is a review of selected cases relevant to adults who have learning disabilities.

## Southeastern Community College v. Davis, 442 U.S. 397 (99 S. Ct. 1979)

This case focused on the issue of reasonable accommodations. A student with a hearing impairment, who was dependent on lip reading, requested that the nursing school she attended waive "practical" course requirements and provide accommodations, such as having a professor with her when working with a patient. The court upheld the school's claim that the ability to hear speech was a necessary qualification for a nurse, and that the accommodations requested would be "substantial" and fall under the category of "undue financial or administrative burden."

## Salvador v. Bell, 622 F. Supp. 438 (N.D. Ill. 1985), aff'd 800 F. 2d 97 (7th Cir. 1986)

The legal issue focused on whether a university discriminated against a student with a disability by failing to provide academic accommodations. In this case, the student failed to inform the university of his learning disability or the need for specific modifications. The court ruled that the university's actions were not discriminatory and did not violate the individual's rights, since the university was not informed that the individual had a learning disability.

## United States v. Board of Trustees for the University of Alabama, 408 F. 2d 740 (11th Cir. 1990)

The legal issue focused on the provision of auxiliary aids, such as interpreters, to students with disabilities. The court ruled that the university could not deny these aids, even in cases where students were able to pay and not in need of fiinancial assistance. The university was obligated to provide auxiliary aids and could not use "undue financial burden" as a criterion to deny this support.

## Wynne v. Tufts University School of Medicine,
## 932 F. 2d 119 (1st Cir. Boston 1990)

The legal issue focused on a student's claim that Tufts discriminated against him on the basis of his disability. The student alleged he had a learning disability and requested that the medical school change the test format to accommodate it. The question was whether he notified the school of his disability and requested accommodations before failing courses. The student claimed that he had difficulty with multiple-choice tests, having failed them several times.

At the end of his first year, he failed eight of the fifteen courses. Tufts arranged for neuropsychological testing (no diagnosis of dyslexia or a learning disability was made) and allowed him to repeat the first-year program. The school also provided the following help: special tutoring in failed courses, the use of note takers, and help with study skills. After failing one course for the third time (biochemistry), he was dismissed from the medical school. He filed suit based on the claim that a different test format (oral examination) would have allowed him to demonstrate his knowledge of the material. The District Court granted judgment in Tufts' favor. The case was appealed, at which time the court again ruled in favor of Tufts. It was decided that the student did not satisfy the criteria as an "otherwise qualified" person under Section 504. The court concluded that the medical school did consider alternative means for testing but decided, first, that the biochemistry course was essential to the curriculum and, second, that the multiple-choice format was the "fairest way" to test mastery of that subject. Any changes would have lowered academic standards and required substantial program alterations.

## Stutts v. Freeman, as Chairman of the Board of Directors of the
## Tennessee Valley Authority, 694 F. 2d 666 (11th Cir. 1983)

The legal issue focused on whether a written test used for job entry discriminated against an individual who had dyslexia. In this case, an individual's application to enter a program to become a heavy-equipment operator was denied, based solely on a low score on the entry test. The court ruled for the plaintiff, stating that in choosing a test as the sole hiring criterion, the Tennessee Valley Authority discriminated against a person with a disability.

## Di Pompo v. West Point Military Academy, 708 F. Supp. 540 (S.D. N.Y. 1989), 770 F. Supp. 887 (S.D. N.Y. 1991)

An individual who had dyslexia was denied application for a firefighting job because his reading score fell below the twelfth-grade level. The question centered on whether he could perform the duties "safely and efficiently" in spite of his low score and reading difficulty. The court upheld the Academy's claim in ruling that reading was essential to meeting the requirements of the job. Even if accommodations were provided, the individual's disability was considered to pose a hazard to the safety of himself and others.

## Dinsmore v. Charles C. Pugh and the Regents of the University of California, Berkeley (1990)

The legal issue focused on whether an institution was responsible for the decision of a professor. In this case, a professor refused to provide a student with dyslexia with additional time to complete a mathematics examination. After the university's intervention was unsuccessful, the student filed suit. The case was settled out of court. As part of the settlement, the university developed a comprehensive policy to accommodate the academic needs of students with disabilities.

## Elizabeth Guckenberger et al. v. Boston University et al., 957 F. Supp. 306, 327 (D. Mass. 1997)

This class action suit was brought by students with learning disorders (ADHD, ADD, learning disabilities) against Boston University. The class claimed that the university's actions were discriminatory and in violation of the Americans with Disabilities Act, the Rehabilitation Act, and state law. The class claimed that the university (1) established unreasonable eligibility criteria to qualify as a disabled student, (2) failed to provide reasonable procedures to review a student's request for accommodations, (3) did not give advance warning to students regarding changes in accommodation policy, and (4) instituted an across-the-board policy denying course substitutions in foreign language and mathematics.

The following summarizes the court's ruling:

1. "Federal law prohibits private and public universities, colleges, and post-secondary educational institutions from discriminating against students with specific learning disabilities."
2. Boston University did not show that the eligibility criteria it used were "necessary to the provision of educational services or reasonable accommodations."
3. Boston University did not give advance warning regarding changes in policy and in so doing delayed or denied reasonable accommodations.
4. Boston University did not provide adequate accommodations for students who had learning disabilities and who had difficulty learning a foreign language.

The court supported the university on the following issues:

1. The class complaint about the mathematics requirement was dismissed.
2. The university was given the opportunity to reconsider the foreign language requirement.
3. The court ruled that a university is not required to modify requirements or provide accommodations that compromise the academic standards of the institution.

This case has been settled in the courts. The decision will have a significant impact on institutions of higher education, as well as on students who have learning disabilities.

## Bartlett v. New York State Board of Law Examiners
## United States Court of Appeals, 156 F. 3d 321 (2nd Cir. N.Y. 1998)

The suit was brought by Marilyn J. Bartlett, a law school graduate, against the New York State Board of Law Examiners. Dr. Bartlett applied for the bar examination as a reading disabled candidate on three or four occasions. She requested the following accommodations: extended time to take the test and permission to tape-record her essays and to circle multiple-choice answers in the test booklet. The Board denied these requests, claiming that according to their expert opinion, she did not meet the criteria for a reading disability. Dr. Bartlett took the examination four times without accommodations and failed each time.

In 1993, after the Board again denied her application for accommodations, Dr. Bartlett brought a complaint against the Law Board, claiming that its decision violated the Americans with Disabilities Act and the Rehabilitation Act. In the suit, she asked for reasonable accommodations and compensatory damages.

An agreement was reached between the parties. Dr. Bartlett was permitted the following accommodations for the July 1993 bar examination: time-and-a-half for the New York portion of the test, the use of an amanuensis to read test questions and record responses, and the option to mark answers to multiple-choice questions in a question book rather than using the computerized answer sheet. The parties also agreed that if Dr. Bartlett passed the examination, the results would not be certified unless she won the lawsuit. Dr. Bartlett failed the examination despite the accommodations.

The Board continued to deny Dr. Bartlett's request for accommodations. They cited the opinion of their expert who claimed she did not have dyslexia or a reading disability. This opinion was based on her scores on two subtests of a standardized reading test, which fell above the 30th percentile.

The Court agreed with Dr. Bartlett's experts who claimed that she had an "automaticity and a reading rate problems." The Court concluded that clinical judgment must be considered in the decision process, as "a reading disability is not quantifiable merely in test scores."

The Court held that Dr. Bartlett is disabled under the meaning of the Americans with Disabilities Act and Section 504 of the Rehabilitation Act. As such, the New York State Board of Law was considered to be in violation of these statutes. The Court ordered accommodations, as "reasonable accommodations will enable her to compete fairly," and compensatory damages. The accommodations included: double time in taking the examination, the use of a computer, permission to circle multiple-choice answers in the examination booklet, and large print on the New York State and Multistate Bar Examination.

This landmark case is one of the first on an appeal level that addresses the impact of the law on professional licensing organizations. The Court's ruling does provide significant support for individuals who have learning disabilities. With increased numbers of individuals with learning disabilities completing professional degrees, we have yet to see how the law will be interpreted regarding professional standards and job qualifications as well as entitlement to accommodations. This case also highlights the fact that in the field there are no consistently agreed on criteria or cutoff points to diagnose a learning disability.

As in the case against Boston University, policy will be determined on a case-by-case basis. However, this decision will move professional organizations to review standards and policies so that individuals who have learning disabilities have equal opportunities for professional careers.

# Appendix B
## *Related Professionals*

### LEARNING DISABILITIES SPECIALIST

A learning disabilities specialist is a special educator trained to work with individuals with learning disabilities. He or she has a degree in special education, which can be obtained at the bachelors, masters, and doctoral levels. Most learning disabilities specialists have, at the minimum, a master's degree. Most states require a teaching certificate to work in the public schools. Currently, there are no state certification requirements or established criteria for specialists working with adults.

A learning disabilities specialist may work in schools, clinics, community agencies, private practice, or any other setting to provide instruction to individuals with learning disabilities. Instruction is provided individually or in groups. He or she is trained to deal with all aspects of the curriculum, which includes the range of academic skills, such as reading, writing, and mathematics, as well as strategies to facilitate learning. A learning disabilities specialist is also trained to assess the achievement of academic skills and strategies. Some specialists are trained to assess cognitive skills as well.

### READING SPECIALIST

A reading specialist is an educator who is trained in the teaching of reading. He or she may have training in elementary, secondary, or special education, in addition to specific training in the teaching of reading. Generally, a degree in reading is obtained at the masters or doctoral level. A reading specialist provides literacy instruction for those with and without disabilities. A reading specialist may work in schools, clinical settings, or in private practice, diagnosing and treating reading problems in children, adolescents, and adults. As is the case with learning disabilities special-

ists, there are no state certification requirements or established criteria for specialists working with adults.

## PSYCHOLOGIST

A psychologist is trained to evaluate children and adults and treat those with psychological problems. Typically, it is a psychologist who administers cognitive and projective tests (in some cases, academic achievement tests as well). A psychologist also provides counseling, psychotherapy, and may serve as a consultant to other professionals. Within the field there are several different areas of specialization, such as school psychology, clinical psychology, developmental psychology, and neuropsychology. Most practicing psychologists have earned doctoral degrees in psychology. A psychologist can work in a school setting with a master's degree in school psychology and state certification. Psychologists with a doctoral degree must be licensed to practice.

## SPEECH-LANGUAGE PATHOLOGIST

A speech-language pathologist evaluates and treats children and adults with speech and/or language problems. A master's degree is needed to work as a clinician in a hospital, school, or private office setting. A teaching certificate issued by the state in which he or she is teaching is needed to work within the public school system. Speech language pathologists with doctoral degrees may be engaged in research or teaching at the college or graduate-school level.

A speech-language pathologist is trained to work with a range of developmental and acquired speech or language problems. Speech problems include difficulty with fluency, voice, or articulation of sounds and words. Language problems include difficulty at the receptive and expressive levels, which involves comprehension and expression of language. Intervention is provided individually or, in some cases, in small groups.

## PSYCHIATRIST

A psychiatrist is a physician who is trained to diagnose and treat psychosocial or psychiatric problems in children and adults. A psychiatrist

has a medical degree and residency training in an area of specialization, such as child and adolescent psychiatry, addiction psychiatry, or forensic or geriatric psychiatry.

A psychiatrist works with individuals who have developmental or psychosocial problems, such as poor social skills or limited self-esteem, and psychiatric disorders such as depression, bipolar disorder, anxiety, and attention-deficit/hyperactivity disorder. Treatment involves the use of medication, psychotherapy, or a multimodal approach.

## NEUROLOGIST

A neurologist is a physician who is trained to diagnose and treat developmental and/or acquired neurological problems in children and adults. A neurologist has a medical degree, followed by residency training in an area of specialization, such as pediatric neurology, electrophysiology, stroke, or epilepsy.

A neurologist diagnoses problems related to trauma, brain injury, degenerative diseases of the central nervous system, epilepsy, and attention-deficit/hyperactivity disorder. Treatment includes medication, referral for surgery, and rehabilitative approaches to trauma or disease.

# Appendix C
## *Selected Tests Used for Older Adolescents and Adults*

### TESTS TAPPING
### A RANGE OF COGNITIVE ABILITIES

Bender Visual Motor Gestalt Test (Bender, 1928), ages 5 to adult

Detroit Tests of Learning Aptitude–Adult (Hammill and Bryant, 1992), ages 16 to adult

Wechsler Adult Intelligence Scale–III (Wechsler, 1997), ages 16 to 89 years

Woodcock-Johnson Psychoeducational Battery–R, Tests of Cognitive Ability (Woodcock and Johnson, 1989), ages 2 to adult

### TESTS TAPPING
### LANGUAGE AND AUDITORY ABILITIES

Boston Naming Test (Kaplan, Goodglass, Weintraub, 1983), ages 5 to adult

Clinical Evaluation of Language Fundamentals–3 (Semel, Wiig, Secord, 1995), ages 6 to 21 years, 11 months

Comprehensive Test of Phonological Processing (Wagner, Torgesen, Rashotte, 1999), ages 5 to 24 years, 11 months

Goldman-Fristoe-Woodcock Auditory Skills Battery (Goldman, Fristoe, Woodcock, 1976), children and adults

Lindamood Auditory Conceptualization Test, Rev. Ed. (Lindamood and Lindamood, 1979), all ages

Test of Adolescent and Adult Language–3 (Hammill, Brown, Larsen, Wiederholt, 1994), ages 12 to 24 years, 11 months

# TESTS TAPPING
# PSYCHOLOGICAL/EMOTIONAL FUNCTIONING

Rorschach Technique (Rorschach, 1945), children and adults

Thematic Apperception Test (Murray and Bellak, 1973), children and adults

# TESTS TAPPING
# ACADEMIC ABILITIES AND ACHIEVEMENT

Nelson-Denny Reading Test (Brown, Fishco, and Hanna, 1981), ages 16 to adult

Scholastic Abilities Test for Adults (Bryant et al., 1991), ages 16 to adult

Stanford Diagnostic Mathematics Test, 4th ed. (Karlsen and Gardner, 1995) grades 1 to 13

Stanford Diagnostic Reading Test, 4th ed. (Karlsen and Gardner, 1995), Grades 1 to 13

Wechsler Individual Achievement Test (1992), ages 5 to 19 years

Wide Range Achievement Test–3 (Jastak and Wilkinson, 1993), ages 5 to 75 years

Woodcock-Johnson Psychoeducational Battery–R, (Woodcock and Johnson, 1989), ages 2 to adult

Woodcock Reading Mastery Tests–R (Woodcock, 1994) ages 5 to adult

# Appendix D
## Professional Organizations and Agencies

## ORGANIZATIONS

The following directory lists, in alphabetical order, the names, addresses, and a brief description of organizations that might be useful for the adult with learning disabilities or attention-deficit/hyperactivity disorder.

**American Psychological Association (APA)**
750 First St. NE, Washington, DC 20002
This organization represents professionals in psychology.

**American Rehabilitation Counseling Association**
5999 Stevenson Ave., Alexandria, VA 22304
This organization represents professional rehabilitation counselors.

**American Speech-Language-Hearing Association (ASHLA)**
10801 Rockville Pike, Rockville, MD 20852
This organization is a certifying body for speech-language pathologists and audiologists, as well as an accrediting agency for college and university programs in speech-language pathology/audiology.

**Attention Deficit Disorder Association (ADDA)**
P.O. Box 972, Mentor, OH 44061
This organization provides educational resources to individuals and support organizations.

**Children and Adults with Attention Deficit Disorder (CH.A.D.D.)**
499 NW 70th Ave., Suite 308, Plantation, FL 33317
A parent-based organization that disseminates information on attention-deficit disorders.

**Clearinghouse on Adult Education and Literacy**
U.S. Department of Education
400 Maryland Ave. SW, Washington, DC 20202
A clearinghouse that provides resources in adult education and helps to connect individuals with the Office of Adult Education within their state.

**Council for Exceptional Children**
1920 Association Dr., Reston, VA 22091
An organization of special educators, related professionals, students, parents, and others who are interested in the education and welfare of individuals with special needs.

**Council for Learning Disabilities**
P.O. Box 40303, Overland Park, KS 66204
A national organization of professionals who work with individuals with learning disabilities.

**HEATH Resource Center**
1 Dupont Circle, Suite 800, Washington, DC 20036
This national clearinghouse disseminates information about postsecondary education for individuals with disabilities.

**International Dyslexia Association**
8600 LaSalle Rd., Suite 382, Towson, MD 21286-2044
An international organization dedicated to the study and treatment of dyslexia.

**International Reading Association**
800 Barksdale Rd., Newark, DE 19711
An organization of professionals and others interested in promoting high levels of literacy and literacy instruction.

**Learning Disabilities Association of America**
4156 Library Road, Pittsburgh, PA 15234
A national organization of parents, adults, and professionals who work to meet the needs of individuals with learning disabilities and their families. This is done through advocacy and the sponsoring of legislation and regulations.

**Literacy Volunteers of America, Inc.**

57195 Widewaters Parkway, Syracuse, NY 13214

A national organization that works to alleviate illiteracy through a network of community volunteer literacy programs.

**National Center for Law and Learning Disabilities (NCLLD)**

P.O. Box 368, Cabin John, MD 20818

This organization seeks to promote understanding of learning disabilities, attention-deficit/hyperactivity disorder, and related conditions. This is accomplished through education, advocacy, analysis of legal issues, and policy recommendations.

**National Center for Learning Disabilities**

99 Park Ave., New York, NY 10016

A national organization dedicated to helping children with learning disabilities through such activities as raising public awareness and understanding and providing national computerized information about referral, educational programs, and legislative advocacy.


# GOVERNMENT OFFICES THAT PROVIDE INFORMATION ABOUT THE AMERICANS WITH DISABILITIES ACT, SECTION 504, IDEA AND EQUAL EMPLOYMENT OPPORTUNITIES ISSUES

**Department of Justice**

Office of Americans with Disabilities Act

Civil Rights Division

P.O. Box 66118, Washington, DC 20035

The Department provides information regarding "public accommodation" issues, specified under the Americans with Disabilities Act.

**Equal Opportunity Employment Commission**

1801 L St. NW, Washington, DC 20507

This office provides information about discrimination and issues in employment settings, for example, job-application procedures, hiring, discharge, job training.

## Office of Civil Rights
U.S. Department of Education
400 Maryland Ave. SW, Washington, DC 20202
> This office provides information on issues regarding Section 504, and IDEA as they apply to the rights of individuals in public school settings.

## President's Committee on Employment of People with Disabilities
1331 F St. NW, Washington, DC 20004

# Appendix E
## *Guides for College Planning*

**Directory of Educational Facilities for Learning Disabled Students**
Learning Disabilities Association of America
4156 Library Rd., Pittsburgh, PA 15234
   The directory provides information on facilities that accept and provide education to individuals with learning disabilities.

**Getting LD Students Ready for College**
HEATH Resource Center
1 Dupont Circle NW, Washington, DC 20036
   The guide lists skills needed and steps to take to prepare high school
   students with learning disabilities for college.

**K & W Guide to Colleges for the Learning Disabled**
Educators Publishing Service, Inc.
31 Smith Pl., Cambridge, MA 02138
   The guide provides a list of colleges that offer services for students
   with learning disabilities.

**Lovejoy's College Guide for the Learning Disabled**
Special Needs Project
1482 East Valley Rd., Santa Barbara, CA 93108
   The guide provides information about colleges and universities, predominantly four-year institutions.

**Peterson's Colleges with Programs for**
**Students with Learning Disabilities**
Peterson's
202 Carnegie Center, P.O. Box 2123, Princeton, NJ 08543
   The directory provides information about more than 900 two- and
   four-year colleges that offer a range of services to students with learning disabilities.

# Appendix F
## *Professional Journals*

### *Journal of Learning Disabilities*
Pro-Ed
8700 Shoal Creek Blvd., Austin TX 78757
(800) 897-3202; (800) Fx PROED (Fax)
   A multidisciplinary publication on learning disabilities that presents articles on research, theory, and instruction.

### *Learning Disability Quarterly*
Council for Learning Disabilities
P.O. Box 40303, Overland Park, KS 66204
(913) 492-8755
   Presents research on learning disabilities.

### *Reading Research Quarterly*
International Reading Association
800 Barksdale Rd., P.O. Box 8139
Newark, DE 19714
   Presents research on reading.

### *Intervention in School and Clinic*
Pro-Ed
8700 Shoal Creek Blvd., Austin, TX 78757
(800) 897-3202; (800) Fx PROED (Fax)
   Presents articles on intervention used by practitioners in both classrooms and clinics.

### *Remedial and Special Education*
Pro-Ed
8700 Shoal Creek Blvd., Austin TX 78757
(800) 897-3202; (800) Fx PROED (Fax)
   Presents articles on research and instruction.

### LD Research and Practice
Council for Exceptional Children
1920 Association Dr., Reston, VA 22091
(703) 620-3660; (800) 328-0272

Presents current research in the field appropriate for researchers and instructors.

### Journal of Adolescent and Adult Literacy
International Reading Association
800 Barksdale Rd., P.O. Box 8139
Newark, DE 19714

Presents articles on research and instruction of literacy for adolescents and adults.

### Annals of Dyslexia
The International Dyslexia Association
Chester Building, Suite 382, 8600 La Salle Rd.
Towson, MD 22044

Interdisciplinary journal presenting research, reviews, and instructional recommendations related to reading disability.

### LD: A Multidisciplinary Journal
LD Association of America
4156 Library Rd., Pittsburgh, PA 15234
(412) 341-1515

A multidisciplinary journal providing articles on research, theory, and instructional trends related to learning disabilities.

# Glossary

**Accommodations**  Modifications or adjustments within an educational or work program to meet the needs of individuals with learning and other disabilities. Accommodations are mandated by Section 504 of the Rehabilitation Act and the Americans with Disabilities Act.

**Achievement level**  Level of an individual's performance, as measured by tests within the academic areas, such as reading or mathematics.

**Achievement test**  A test that measures the degree to which an individual has acquired information or skills, usually as a result of instruction.

**Americans with Disabilities Act (ADA)**  Federal legislation that sets standards that prohibit discrimination in both public and private programs and facilities.

**Assistive technological devices**  Technological implements (any item, piece of equipment, or product system) used to help individuals with disabilities compensate for their difficulties.

**Attention-deficit/hyperactivity disorder (ADHD)**  A neurologically based disorder characterized by inattention, impulsivity, and hyperactivity. ADHD is defined by and included in the *Diagnostic and Statistical Manual of Mental Disorders,* fourth edition (American Psychiatric Association).

**Attribution theory**  A theory that explains how interpretations of personal experience color or influence the development of motivation and self-esteem.

**Attribution**  The way one interprets the causes of his or her successes or failures.

**Auditory perception**  the ability to recognize and interpret information that one hears.

**Automaticity**  The stage in learning that requires little conscious effort.

**Auxiliary aids**  Supports that enable individuals to compensate for their disability. For individuals with learning disabilities, auxiliary aids might include reading machines, books on tape, calculators, note takers.

**Background knowledge**    Information that an individual stores in memory. This includes educationally related facts, and information gained from experience, as well as specific information about a subject area or a reading selection.

**Basic skills instruction**    Instruction in the rudiments of reading, writing, or mathematics.

**Behavioral management**    A technique used to strengthen positive behavior while decreasing negative behavior. This technique applies the concept of operant conditioning that is part of behavioral psychology.

**Brain electrical mapping**    (BEAM) A procedure that uses computers to map electrical brain waves.

**Carl D. Perkins Vocational and Applied Technology Education Act Amendments**    (Public Law 101-392) Federal legislation that provides access to vocational educational programs and mandates transitional services at the secondary and postsecondary levels.

**Central nervous system**    The organic system that includes the brain and the spinal cord.

**Central nervous system dysfunction**    A disorder resulting from impairment of brain function.

**Cerebral hemispheres**    The two halves of the brain (right and left hemispheres), which are made up of the frontal, temporal, occipital, and parietal lobes.

**Chunking strategy**    Grouping or clustering information together as an aid to storage and recall.

**Cloze procedure**    A testing procedure or instructional format that involves the deletion of words from text and the insertion of blank spaces.

**Cognitive abilities**    A general term that includes the ability to receive, process, reason, and analyze information, and use critical judgment.

**Cognitive instruction**    Instruction in the development of knowledge and strategy use, geared to helping the individual develop a more active approach to organizing new information and retrieving stored facts.

**Collaboration**    The combined efforts of two or more professionals working together to effect an educational or work goal.

**Comorbidity**    The presence of more than one disorder in the same individual. For example, attention-deficit/hyperactivity disorder and learning disabilities are often comorbid conditions.

**Compensatory instruction**    Instruction aimed at developing coping strategies so that tasks can be performed more effectively.

**Correlation**  The relationship between two scores or measures, or the tendency of one score or measure to vary concomitantly with the other.

**Criterion referenced test**  A test that measures an individual's achievement in specific skill areas.

**Curriculum-based assessment**  Assessment that measures an individual's performance on an academic task or within a subject area of the curriculum. These measures are repeated to determine progress in these areas.

**Declarative knowledge**  An individual's knowledge base; what he or she knows.

**Diagnostic test**  A test used to diagnose specific areas of strength or weakness in a skill area, such as reading or mathematics.

**The Diagnostic and Statistical Manual of Mental Disorders, Fourth Edition (DSM-IV)**  The classification system developed by the American Psychiatric Association, used by mental health professionals to classify disorders of children and adults.

**Discrepancy formula**  A mathematical formula used to quantify the difference between ability and achievement; one of the methods used to diagnose a learning disability.

**Distractibility**  Difficulty sustaining attention, focusing on a task, and organizing tasks and activities.

**Dynamic assessment**  An approach to testing that evaluates an individual's performance and potential for learning. Interactive techniques are used to determine the conditions under which an individual might learn a skill more effectively.

**Dyscalculia**  Difficulty learning and using mathematics.

**Dysgraphia**  Difficulty performing the motor movements needed for handwriting; extreme difficulty with handwriting.

**Dyslexia**  A type of learning disability characterized by extreme difficulty learning to read and write, despite conventional instruction and adequate intelligence and not explainable by other conditions or disabilities.

**Eligibility criteria**  Standards used to determine whether a student has a learning disability or other disability in order to be eligible for accommodations or services.

**Emotional functioning**  Feelings and sensitivities about oneself, such as self-worth, self-esteem, and self-reliance.

**Entitlement**  Modifications and services allowed to individuals with disabilities, as set forth in the Individuals with Disabilities Education Act, the Rehabilitation Act, and Americans with Disabilities Act.

**Episodic memory**    Stored information that includes temporal-spatial (time and space) experiences and autobiographical events in one's past.

**Executive function**    A component of the information processing system. The executive function is a hypothesized manager that takes control, monitors, and coordinates an individual's learning and recall.

**Expressive language disorder**    Difficulty expressing language on the verbal or written level.

**External motivation**    A drive to succeed that is motivated by the need to please or perform for others.

**Functional skills instruction**    Instruction in survival skills aimed to equip the individual to manage the activities of daily living.

**Grade equivalent**    The grade level for which a specific score is the real or estimated average.

**Guided learning**    A dynamic technique that involves observing how an individual responds to instruction, then guiding the individual to use strategies and to learn a task or skill.

**Health Research Extension Act, Pl 99-158**    The Act that mandated the development of an Interagency Committee on Learning Disabilities.

**Hyperactivity**    A condition characterized by excessive fidgeting and motor activity.

**IDEA**    Acronym for Individuals with Disabilities Education Act.

**Impulsivity**    Difficulty planning and initiating thoughtful behavior before acting.

**Individualized education program (IEP)**    A written plan, mandated by IDEA, that outlines the education for an individual student with disabilities.

**Individuals with Disabilities Education Act (IDEA)**    The federal law that mandates a free, appropriate, public education for students with disabilities.

**Informal test**    A non-standardized test that can be teacher-made or commercially prepared.

**Information-processing approach**    This approach looks at the steps and activities the human mind takes in processing, storing, retrieving, and expressing information.

**Instructional reading level**    The level at which a student can read with approximately 95 percent accuracy in decoding and approximately 75 percent accuracy in comprehension. This is the level of material commonly used to teach word-recognition skills.

**Intelligence test**    A standardized test that measures both verbal and non-verbal abilities. These abilities make up what is considered intellectual functioning.

**Intelligence quotient (IQ)**   A measure of ability, taking into account the combined scores on an intelligence test and one's age.

**Interactive approaches**   Instructional approaches that utilize teacher and student or peer and student. These approaches are geared to the development of strategy use through the use of modeling and feedback by the teacher or peer.

**Intrinsic motivation**   A drive to succeed that is motivated by one's own needs and goals.

**Learned helplessness**   A trait characterized by an inability to take responsibility for one's actions. This shows up as passivity and dependence on others.

**Learning disabilities**   An umbrella term that encompasses a cluster of disorders or problems that affect different areas of cognitive, academic, and psychosocial functioning.

**Literacy**   Defined by the national Literacy Act (1991) as an individual's ability to read, write, and speak English, and compute and solve problems at levels of proficiency necessary to function on the job and in society and achieve one's goals, and develop one's knowledge and potential.

**Long-term memory**   Information that is permanently stored. Long-term memory has an unlimited capacity and time frame. This storage center is part of the information-processing approach.

**Magnetic resonance imaging (MRI)**   A neuroimaging device based on magnetic fields that displays images of parts of the human anatomy on a video screen.

**Metacognition**   Knowledge about oneself as a learner. This knowledge is needed to control how we learn and to employ task-appropriate strategies.

**Metacognitive theory**   A theory that identifies metacognitive insight, executive control, and strategy use as essential variables needed for processing and storing information and performing a range of activities.

**Metamemory**   Knowledge about one's own memory abilities. This knowledge is needed to control memroy functions and to employ task-appropriate strategies.

**Methylphenidate (Ritalin)**   A stimulant drug that is used for treatment of attention-deficit/hyperactivity disorder.

**Multimodal approach**   A comprehensive treatment approach that combines different therapies, such as the use of psychotherapy and medication to treat ADHD.

**National Institute of Child Health and Human Development**   One of sixteen institutes within the National Institutes of Health, committed to the study of learning disabilities.

**National Joint Committee on Learning Disabilities (NJCLD)**   An organization that includes representatives from different professional organizations and disciplines involved with learning disabilities.

**Neurology**   A medical specialty concerned with the diagnosis and treatment of developmental and acquired problems of the central nervous system.

**Neurons**   Nerve cells.

**Neuropsychological assessment**   A traditional assessment approach that develops a profile of behaviors, abilities, and skills. The neuropsychological assessment is used primarily to identify problems resulting from known brain injury and developmental delays, and to collect clinical data.

**Neurotransmitter**   Chemicals responsible for transmitting messages from one brain cell to another.

**Nontricyclic antidepressants**   A class of drugs used for treatment of attention-deficit/hyperactivity disorder.

**Norms**   Statistics that describe the performance of individuals or groups in a standardization sample. Norms are considered to be representative of the larger population, such as college students nationwide. Percentile, grade, and age are the most common types of norms.

**Percentile**   A score that falls within a distribution or scale of 100. For example, a score in the 75th percentile indicates that 75 percent of the cases fall below this number or percentile.

**Psychotherapy**   A therapeutic approach in the treatment of psychological disorders.

**One-on-one correspondence**   A term used in mathematics to describe the matching of an element of a set to one element of a second set.

**Optical character recognition (OCR) systems**   Reading machines.

**Perceptual disorder**   A disorder that interferes with the ability to perceive and process information received through the auditory, visual, tactile, or kinesthetic channels.

**Perceptual-motor**   Information received through the auditory or visual channel and perceived, integrated, and expressed through a motor activity.

**Performance-based assessment**   A method of assessing individuals by observing and evaluating their performance in an academic or work setting.

**Perseveration**   The behavior of being locked into producing the same response again and again.

**Phoneme**   The smallest unit of meaningful sound; the fundamental element of language.

**Phonic decoding**   Determining the pronunciation of a written word by applying sound to symbol.

**Phonological awareness**   Recognition of the sounds of language; an understanding that speech can be separated into syllables and sounds.

**Phonological blending**   Synthesizing or blending the phonemes in a word.

**Phonological processing**   The ability to identify, interpret, discriminate, organize, store, and retrieve the sounds of language.

**Plasticity of the brain**   The brain's ability to compensate for loss of function.

**Portfolio assessment**   An assessment approach that uses an individual's portfolio of work from school or work or both. This material is evaluated and analyzed over a period of time.

**Positron emission tomography (PET)**   A procedure that measures metabolic activity of the brain.

**Pragmatics**   The ability to use language appropriately in a social context; the social customs involved in language use.

**Procedural knowledge**   An individual's knowledge concerning the steps needed to perform a task.

**Process approach to writing**   Approach that views writing as a multiple-step process that moves through the stages of prewriting, drafting, editing, revising, and sharing.

**Protective factors**   Life situations and events that can enhance the chance of a positive outcome, despite elements of risk.

**Psychoeducational assessment**   A traditional assessment approach that develops a profile of behaviors, abilities, and skills.

**Psychological processing disorders**   A phrase in the federal definition of learning disabilities that refers to disorders of visual or auditory perception, memory, and/or language.

**Public Law 94-142**   The Education for All Handicapped Children Act, landmark federal legislation passed in 1975. This law guarantees a free, appropriate public education to children with disabilities. The law was redefined in 1990 and again in 1997. In 1990 it was renamed the Individuals with Disabilities Education Act.

**Range**   The difference between the lowest and highest score on a test.

**Rating scales**   A measurement tool used by parents, teachers, or informants to rank an individual's behavior.

**Raw score**   In most cases, the number of correct answers on a test.

**Reasonable accommodations**   Section 504 of the Rehabilitation Act and ADA includes this phrase, which refers to adjustments made in an academic or work setting for individuals with disabilities.

**Receptive language disorder**   Difficulty processing or comprehending language.

**The Rehabilitation Act**   Federal legislation that protects the civil rights of individuals of all ages who have disabilities.

**Rehearsal strategy**   A strategy that involves reviewing or repeating information as an aid to storage and recall.

**Reliability**   The degree to which a test provides consistent results. Reliability involves factors such as dependability, stability, and relative freedom from errors of measurement.

**Remedial instruction**   Instruction aimed at improving areas of weakness typically in reading, writing, and mathematics.

**Resource room**   A room within a school where instruction is delivered by a special education teacher to a child or small group of children with special learning needs.

**Retrieval**   Recall of information from memory.

**Risk factors**   Life situations, events, or circumstances that can have a negative impact on one's life.

**Scaffolded instruction**   Teaching approach in which the teacher provides support which is gradually withdrawn as the learners demonstrate mastery of new skills and strategies.

**Schemas**   Clusters or files of information stored in long-term memory.

**School-to-Work Opportunities Act**   Federal legislation that provides support for individuals preparing for the workplace. Programs include a school- or work-based learning component, as well as other supportive activities.

**Self-determination**   An individual's ability and willingness to assume responsibility for defining his or her own goals as well as accepting responsibility for accomplishments and setbacks.

**Self-esteem**   Feelings of self-worth and self-confidence.

**Self-regulated learner**   A motivated problem solver who is actively engaged and has control over his or her own learning; a learner who has acquired strategies, applies them, and modifies them to accomplish learning tasks.

**Semantic memory**   Stored information that includes a thesaurus, language symbols, rules, and generalizations.

**Sensory register**   The initial stage in the memory system. Sensory signals are perceived and briefly analyzed before they are sent to short-term memory. This center is part of the information-processing approach.

**Short-term (working) memory**   Information from the sensory register is consciously processed within working memory. This information is temporarily stored, then either transferred to long term memory or displaced by new stimuli. This storage center is part of the information-processing approach.

**Sight words**   Printed words recognized automatically/instantly, primarily by their visual configuration.

**Social judgment**   Ability to judge feelings, moods, and attitudes of others.

**Social perception**   The ability to perceive and understand social cues and situations as well as the feelings of others.

**Social skills deficit**   Deficit that interferes with the ability to judge, perceive, and interpret social cues and enact an appropriate social response.

**Soft neurological signs**   Non-focal neurological signs, such as awkwardness of gait. Neurologists associate these signs with mild underlying neurological dysfunction.

**Speech synthesizer**   A computerized voice output system that can read back text displayed on the computer screen.

**Standard deviation**   A measure of the variability of a set of scores or the degree to which the scores cluster around the mean.

**Standard score**   A statistically "transformed" raw score, such as a scaled score. Standard scores help in test interpretation and in making comparisons across tests.

**Standardized test**   A test that must be administered, interpreted and scored according to prescribed conditions (such as time) and rules.

**Stanine**   A scale with values from 1 to 9, with a mean of 5 and a standard deviation of 2.

**Strategy**   A problem-solving behavior that involves effort, planning, and monitoring.

**Structural analysis**   The strategy of identifying words by analyzing word units such as prefixes, suffixes, and root words.

**Support groups**   Groups of individuals that share problems and experiences. The goal is to work out these problems through guidance and the support of others.

**Surveying**   A prereading strategy that involves previewing text by looking at the title, subheadings, pictures, graphs, and words in bold print, and then using that information for predicting and setting the purpose for reading.

**Task analysis**   An instructional approach that breaks an activity down into a sequence of small steps.

**Tech-Prep Act**   Federal legislation that encourages the reorganization of curricula and vocational programs, with the goal of integrating academic and job-related information into the workplace.

**Technology-Related Assistance for Individuals with Disabilities Act Amendments**   Federal legislation that provides discretionary grants to states to assist in the development of programs and financing mechanisms. The goal is to provide technological assistance to individuals with disabilities.

**Temporal processing problem**   The brain's inability to process sensory information that enters the nervous system in rapid succession.

**Transition** Refers to the shift from one educational setting to another or to emergent roles in society.

**Transition planning**   Typically, planning for the move from school to postsecondary school or the workplace, and for role changes in adult life.

**Transition services**   As defined by IDEA, a coordinated set of activities, selected on the basis of the student's needs, preferences, and interests, that promote movement from school to postschool.

**Tricyclic antidepressants**   A class of drugs used for the treatment of attention-deficit/hyperactivity disorder.

**Utah criteria for diagnosis of ADHD**   A rating scale to identify symptoms of attention-deficit/hyperactivity disorder. The scale includes two parts: childhood history and adult diagnostic criteria.

**VAKT approach**   A multisensory approach to the teaching of reading that uses the visual, auditory, kinesthetic, and tactile modalities. Students are taught to identify words by seeing, hearing, and tracing them.

**Validity**   The degree to which the content of a test represents an adequate sampling of the skills or content of an instructional program, or the degree to which the test measures what it is designed to measure.

**Visual perception**   The ability to recognize and interpret information that one sees.

**Visual spatial skills**   The ability to identify, organize, and interpret visual information positioned in space.

**Vocational rehabilitation**   A federal and state program designed to assist individuals with disabilities in obtaining gainful and productive employment that is consistent with their capabilities, interests, resources, priorities, and concerns.

**Word-recognition skills**   Skills used for decoding printed words, including sight word recognition, structural analysis, and phonic decoding.

# References

American Psychiatric Association. 1994. *Diagnostic and statistical manual of mental disorders* (4th ed., rev.). Washington, D.C.

Barkley, R. A., 1990. *Attention-deficit hyperactivity disorder: A handbook for diagnosis and treatment.* New York: Guilford Press.

Bialock, G, and J. R. Patton, 1996. Transition and students with learning disabilities: Creating sound futures. *Journal of Learning Disabilities* 29 (1): 7–16.

Biederman, J., K. Munir, D. Knee, W. Habelow, M. Armentano, S. Autor, S. K. Hoge, and C. Waternaux. 1986. A family study of patients with attention deficit disorder and normal controls. *Journal of Psychiatric Research* 20: 263–74.

Binet, A., and T. Simon, 1905. Méthodes nouvelles pour le diagnostic du niveau intellectual des anormaux. *L'Annee Psychologique* 11: 191–244.

Bradley, W. 1937. The behavior of children receiving benzedrine. *American Journal of Psychiatry* 94: 577–85.

Brinckerhoff, L. 1996. Making the transition to higher education: Opportunities for student empowerment. *Journal of Learning Disabilities* 29: 118–36.

Brinckerhoff, L., S. Shaw, and J. McGuire. 1992. Promoting access, accommodations, and independence for college students with learning disabilities. *Journal of Learning Disabilities* 25: 417–29.

Campione, J. C., and A. Brown. 1978. Toward a theory of intelligence: Contributions from research with retarded children. *Intelligence* 2: 279–304.

Cantwell, D. P. 1996. Attention deficit disorder: A review of the past 10 years. *Journal of the American Academy of Child and Adolescent Psychiatry* 35: 978–87.

Erikson, E. H. 1968. *Identity: Youth and crisis.* New York: Norton.

Faraone, S., and J. Biederman. 1998. Neurobiology of Attention-Deficit Hyperactivity Disorder. *Society of Biological Psychiatry* 44: 951–55.

Feuerstein, R. 1979. *The dynamic assessment of retarded performers: The learning potential assessment device, theory, instruments, and techniques.* Baltimore: University Park Press.

Flavell, J. H. 1970. Developmental studies of mediated memory. In *Advances in child development and behavior.* Ed. H. W. Reese and L. P. Lipsitt. Vol. 5. New York: Academic Press.

Fletcher, J. M., and B. A. Shaywitz. 1996. Attention-deficit/hyperactivity disorder. In *Learning disabilities: Lifelong issues.* Ed. S. C. Cramer and W. Ellis. Baltimore: Paul H. Brookes.

Fletcher, J. M., B. A. Shaywitz, and S. E. Shaywitz. 1994. In *Frames of reference for the assessment of learning disabilities: New views on measurement issues.* Ed. G. Reid Lyon. Baltimore: Paul H. Brookes.

Ganschow, L., J. Coyne, A. W. Parks, and S. J. Antonoff. 1999. A 10-year follow-up survey of programs and services for students with learning disabilities in graduate and professional schools. *Journal of Learning Disabilities* 32(1): 72–84.

Gardner, H. 1993. *Multiple intelligences: The theory in practice.* New York: Basic Books.

Geller, B., and J. Luby. 1997. Child and adolescent bipolar disorder: A review of the past 10 years. *Journal of the American Academy of Child and Adolescent Psychiatry* 36: 1168–76.

Gerber, P. J., R. Ginsberg, and H. Reiff. 1992. Identifying alterable patterns in employment success for highly successful adults with learning disabilities. *Journal of Learning Disabilities* 25: 475–87.

Gerber, P., H. Reiff, and R. Ginsberg. 1996. Reframing the learning disabilities experience. *Journal of Learning Disabilities* 29(1): 98–101.

Kavale, K., and S. Forness. 1996. Social skill deficits and learning disabilities: A meta-analysis. *Journal of Learning Disabilities* 29: 226–37.

Keogh, B. K. 1996. Strategies for implementing policies. In *Learning disabilities: Lifelong issues.* Ed. S. C. Cramer and W. Ellis. Baltimore: Paul H. Brookes.

Keogh, B. K., R. Gallimore, and T. Weisner. 1997. A sociocultural perspective on learning and learning disabilities. *Learning Disabilities Research and Practice* 12: 107–13.

Keogh, B. K., and T. Weisner. 1993. An ecocultural perspective on risk and protective factors in children's development: Implications for learning disabilities. *Learning Disabilities Research and Practice* 8: 3–10.

Licht, B. G. and J. A. Kistner. 1986. Motivational problems of learning disabled children: Individual differences and their implications for treatment. In *Psychological and Educational Perspectives on Learning Disabilities*. Ed. J. K. Torgesen and B. Y. L. Wong. New York: Academic Press.

Lyon, G. R. 1984. *Frames of reference for the assessment of learning disabilities: New views on measurement issues*. Baltimore: Paul H. Brookes.

————. 1991. *Research in learning disabilities* (technical report). Bethesda, MD: National Institute on Child Health and Human Development.

Meichenbaum, D. H. 1997. *Cognitive-behavioral modification: An integrative approach*. New York: Plenum Press.

Meltzer, L. J. 1994. The assessment of learning disabilities: The challenge of evaluating the cognitive strategies and processes underlying learning, In *Frames of reference for the assessment of learning disabilities: New views on measurement issues*. Ed. C. Reid Lyon. Baltimore: Paul H. Brookes.

National Joint Committee on Learning Disabilities. 1994. Collective perspectives on issues affecting learning disabilities. Austin, TX: PRO-ED.

Palincsar, A. S., and A. L. Brown. 1984. Reciprocal teaching of comprehension fostering and comprehension monitoring activities. *Cognition and Instruction* 1: 117–75.

Patton, J., and E. Palloway. 1992. Learning disabilities: The challenges of adulthood. *Journal of Learning Disabilities* 25: 410–29.

Pennington, B. F. 1991. *Diagnosing learning disorders: A neuropsychological framework*. New York: Guilford Press.

Shaywitz, S. 1996. Dyslexia. *Scientific American* 275(5): 98–104.

Spekman, N. J., R. J. Goldberg, and K. L. Herman. 1992. Learning disabled children grow up: A search for factors related to success in the young adult years, *Learning Disabilities Research and Practice* 7: 161–70.

————. 1993. An exploration of risk and resilience in the lives of individuals with learning disabilities. *Learning Disabilities Research and Practice* 8: 11–18.

Spencer, T., J. Biederman, T. Wilens, M. Harding, D. O'Donnell, and S. Griffin. 1996. Pharmacotherapy of attention-deficit hyperactivity disorder across the life cycle. *Journal of the American Academy of Child and Adolescent Psychiatry* 35(4): 409–32.

Sternberg, R. J. 1985. General intellectual ability. In *Human abilities, an information-processing approach*. Ed. R. J. Steinberg. New York: Freeman.

Stone, C. Addison. 1998. The metaphor of scaffolding: Its utility for the field of learning disabilities. *Journal of Learning Disabilities* 31(4): 344–64.

Strauss, A. A., and L. E. Lehtinen. 1947. *Psychopathology and education of the brain injured child.* New York: Grune & Stratton.

Swanson, H. L. 1991. *Handbook on the assessment of learning disabilities: Theory, research & practice.* Texas: PRO-ED.

———. 1993. Learning disabilities from the perspective of cognitive psychology. In *Better understanding learning disabilities: New views from research and their implications for education and public policies.* Ed. G. Reid Lyon, D. B. Gray, J. F. Kavanagh, and N. A. Krasnegor. Baltimore: Paul H. Brookes.

Tallal, P., S. L. Miller, G. Bedi, G. Byma, X. Wang, S. Nagaranjan, C. Schreiner, W. Jenkins, and M. Merzenich. 1996. Language comprehension in language-learning impaired children improved with acoustically modified speech. *Science* 271: 81–84.

Terman, L. 1916. *The measurement of intelligence.* Boston: Houghton-Mifflin.

Vogel, S. A., and P. B. Adelman. 1992. *Success for college students with learning disabilities.* New York: Springer-Verlag.

Vogel, S. A., P. J. Hruby, and P. B. Adelman. 1993. Educational and psychological factors in successful and unsuccessful college students with learning disabilities. *Learning Disabilities Research and Practice* 8(1): 35–43.

Vogel, S., F. Leonard, W. Scales, P. Hayeslip, J. Hermansen, and L. Donnells. 1998. The national learning disabilities data bank: An overview. *Journal of Learning Disabilities* 31(3): 234–47.

Ward, M. F., P. H. Wender, and F. W. Reimherr. 1993. The Wender Utah rating scale: An aid in the retrospective diagnosis of attention deficit hyperactivity disorder, *American Journal of Psychiatry* 150: 885–90.

Wechsler, D. 1939. *Measurement of adult intelligence.* Baltimore: Williams & Wilkins.

Wender, P. H. 1995. *Attention-deficit hyperactivity disorder in adults.* New York: Oxford University Press.

Werner, E. E. 1993. Risk and resilience in individuals with learning disabilities: Lessons learned from the Kauai longitudinal study. *Learning Disabilities Research and Practice* 8(1): 28–34.

# Index

Note: Page numbers in **bold** indicate illustrations.